Psychotherapy with Young People in Care

Whilst there is a wealth of literature on working with children and adolescents, very little focuses on those who are in residential or foster care. *Psychotherapy with Young People in Care* is a practical guide to working with this group from a psychoanalytic therapeutic perspective.

Drawing on the author's years of experience and illustrated with a wealth of clinical examples, as well as a comprehensive glossary, the book tackles those issues most relevant to all those working with children and adolescents:

- The place of psychotherapy in residential / foster care.
- Ethical considerations:
  - Confidentiality
  - Sexual abuse.
- Particular problems faced by young people:
  - ADHD
  - Trauma
  - PTSD.

This refreshing and valuable book is an essential teaching text for all those who work with young people in the care system, including child and adolescent psychotherapists, psychiatrists, clinical psychologists and social workers.

Margaret Hunter is a Child Psychotherapist, with seventeen years' experience of working with children in care. Trained at the Tavistock Clinic, she is now Head of Child Psychotherapy at the Maudsley NHS Trust and continues to work with fostered children at the Integrated Support Programme in Kent. She contributed to the *Handbook of Child and Adolescent Psychotherapy* (Routledge 1999).

This book is dedicated to Norah and Lucius Daly,
my mother and father

Psychotherapy with Young People in Care

Lost and Found

Margaret Hunter

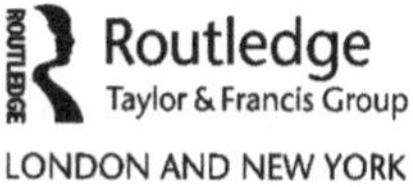

LONDON AND NEW YORK

First published 2001
by Routledge
4 Park Square, Milton Park, Abingdon, Oxon OX14 4RN

Simultaneously published in the USA and Canada
by Taylor & Francis Inc.
605 Third Avenue, New York, NY 10017

Routledge is an imprint of the Taylor & Francis Group, an informa business

Typeset in Times by Keystroke, Jacaranda Lodge, Wolverhampton
Cover design by Louise Page

British Library Cataloguing in Publication Data
A catalogue record for this book is available from the British Library

Library of Congress Cataloging in Publication Data
Hunter, Margaret, 1949–
Psychotherapy with young people in care : lost and found /
Margaret Hunter.
p. cm.
Includes bibliographical references and index.
ISBN 0–415–19190–4 — ISBN 0–415–19191–2 (pbk.)
1. Child psychotherapy—Residential treatment.
2. Child psychotherapy. I. Title.

RJ504.5 .H86 2001
618.92′8914—dc21 00–045706

ISBN 13: 978-0-415-19191-3 (pbk)

Contents

Foreword

This book is about the plight of children who for one reason or another cannot live safely in their own homes. They are 'looked after' by their local authorities, mostly in foster homes and children's homes. Their lives have been severely disrupted; some by tragic loss of parents through death, others through family breakdown and others through sheer abuse and maltreatment. Their predicament, without the sure sense of belonging that most of us have enjoyed with our own parents in our own homes, is in itself precarious. It is made none the more palatable in our contemporary society where we effectively choose to sideline them, overlook or forget them and in too many cases continue to maltreat them. We accommodate them in circumstances that are often poorly resourced and inadequately staffed (with little or no experience or training). We unaccountably and all too often move them from one home to another and we fail to ensure that the education that they receive is sufficiently responsive to their particular needs. It cannot therefore be of surprise that many should have serious mental health problems and that a substantial proportion encounter considerable difficulties, plunged into premature independence, in leaving care.

There are significant moves afoot at present, initiated by the Government, primarily through its 'Quality Protects' programme, to ensure more effective multi-agency management and delivery of services and appropriate assessment, treatment and support for these children. This is all very much to be welcomed. Nevertheless it remains the case that very little has been done, whether in specific research or through clinical studies, to focus on their experience and treatment. There has been in fact a reluctance among psychotherapists to work with such children – generally seen as being poorly motivated, lacking self-observation, prone to acting out and suffering 'external' difficulties in their lives beyond the reach of psychotherapy. Caution has been warned against establishing any psychotherapeutic arrangement with them until the circumstances of their lives have become more settled in 'permanent' placements. The result has been that few such arrangements have been made.

Margaret Hunter, a child psychotherapist who has devoted a great deal of her practice to working with a wide variety of such children, breaks through all this resistance, opening up a realm of therapeutic possibility that is quite inspiring. In this book she draws on her imagination and courage as well as an indispensable knowledge of psychoanalysis and child development. She shows the level of skill and resource that is required to listen to these children, to take the risk of receiving (through her thoughts and her feelings) their experience and to find within them the capacity to bear insight and move beyond the destructive influences of their past lives.

The book is based on her experience of working with eighty children, all in local authority care, mostly in child and family consultation centres and social service departments. Despite the similarities in their circumstances, all present themselves in their own individual ways – some very distracted, impulsive, barely able to make any sustained relationship; others are more stable, capable of symbolic play and ready to draw on their past lives to learn, albeit gradually, from the here-and-now experience of the therapeutic relationship. Margaret Hunter has worked in different ways with these children, some several times a week over five or six years, others more on a short-term assessment basis. Always she has kept in mind the context in which she is working – in a world of social workers, lawyers, foster parents, natural parents and teachers in relation to issues of placement, contact, access and, most disturbingly, child protection. Thirty-two of the children she writes about have been sexually abused, and severely so. Despite the extraordinary intensity of her work with individual children, she never loses sight of her role as a child psychotherapist within the framework of the law and of social responsibility. She faces, for example, the vexed question of confidentiality, holding on as best she can to her respect for the privacy of the child yet acting at times in their best interests, relieving in effect their burden of carrying shameful and intolerable secrets. She also recognises the disarray that can accumulate in the relationships between professionals and agencies, arising as much as anything from the turbulence that resides within the child and within the fragmentation of the child's family.

All of these issues and difficulties come alive in this book which is full of stories, games and pictures that the children tell and play. What is so vivid are their doings and inventions. They occur spontaneously in psychotherapy, in a setting in which feelings can be experienced, memories remembered, thinking made permissible and possible. Margaret Hunter does not regard herself as a teacher, priest or counsellor; her role, she sees, as 'neutral', 'off to one side', not obscured or invaded by other people's agendas, 'getting alongside' the child to allow them to lead, to follow their point of view. None of this is straightforward and she has no illusions about the reality of what actually happens; as she puts it, 'psychotherapy is often a ragbag of loose ends and unanswered questions'. But she never loses sight of her crucial purpose and endeavour: to listen, to contain, to foster thought, to link and piece things together towards self-understanding and ultimately towards different ways of behaving and experiencing the world.

With this at the centre of her mind, she draws close to the poignancy and tragedy of the lives of the children that she helps. She catches the pangs of their longingness ('for what might have been, for what had been, but got lost'), of betrayal and mistrust, of sadness and helplessness. As we read on, we become alarmed by the power of their terror, and of their outrage in the face of abuse and deception. We are appalled by the things that parents have done to them – attempting to drown them, locking them up in cupboards or car boots, hitting them repeatedly, raping them. We come through all of this to an understanding of their fury, their disordered, revengeful behaviour, their frenetic excitements (engendered out of fear and excessive stimulation). We begin to make sense of the way they are, whether it be their uneasy compliance, their constant wariness, their repetitive self-destructiveness or their unremitting attacking, sadistic, and indeed abusive behaviour.

We find out a great deal about them through Margaret Hunter's fine and imaginative observations. The question remains as to what can be done with such a wealth and depth of dreadful experience. It is here that she gives a very convincing account of how she operates and of how child psychotherapists and others closely uninvolved in this field need to develop. It matters first of all that she manages to harness the myriad of images, incidents and feelings into a theoretical framework that makes sense to her. This is of crucial importance since it provides her with her own sense of conceptual coherence. She understands, for example, the pervasive force of primitive unconscious processes such as splitting, projective identification, denial, dissociation. She knows about the bodily preoccupations and sexual theories of children that shape their understanding of adult sexuality, not least sexual abuse. She appreciates the importance of identifications in the way in which children fortify themselves and of repetition compulsion as they are compelled to re-enact their painful past experiences in current relationships and in therapy.

It is perhaps with respect to this last phenomenon that she writes with the greatest clarity and persuasion. For it is here, as she enters into relationships with them, as she opens herself up for engagement with them, that she works emotionally within herself to appreciate the texture of their lostness, their seeking of attachment, their confusion and disappointment, their fear and anger. In her human responses to all of this, through her counter-transference (i.e. what is evoked within her by the expectations, provocations and enactments of her children) she gains a unique understanding of what they have gone through, and what is going on in their lives. At various times, with various children in different circumstances, she writes with remarkable honesty of how she is made to feel – bewildered, unbalanced, ignored, excluded, envious, seduced, excited, bullied, revengeful, hopeless, guilty. None of this gamut of feeling is of course easy to endure but she makes it clear that such experience is essential if the children are to feel understood and the therapist is to make effective contact. She writes that conducting therapy is a 'hazardous venture', the therapist serving as a repository .for memories, receptive to the pain of the children whilst 'dropping one's guard' to think and consider. As she puts it, 'it is their anxiety levels that wear us down' and she emphasises the need for self-awareness and the importance of finding time to disentangle her own feelings from those of the children. She also stresses (as much as she might value the importance of receptivity) the need for the therapist to safeguard her own boundaries, to assert her own right to not be abused and in this way to establish clear structure and order in her sessions. At times, especially with the more frantic and undifferentiated children, she establishes her own firm control, making clear the rules of the game, by dint of her perseverance, her commitment to them.

This book shows us young people who have been lost from the warmth of their families and who have been found through the understanding earned in psychotherapy. At the heart of the book is Margaret Hunter's compassion, vision and toughness. She is fearless in her readiness to engage with the shattered and dislocated lives of the children she works with. She is attentive to detail, sensitive to mood and 'sudden looks'. She shows us quite directly how she 'reads' the symbolism of children's play (their wild cats, their dinosaurs, their disappearing into 'sinking mud') and takes on the different roles that the children require of her in their play. And yet she demonstrates the importance of her training and discipline in exploring her own reactions, questioning herself and steadfastly refusing to placate or retaliate in response to the children's uncertainties, anticipations or provocations.

At a time when, thankfully, there is increasing concern about the lives of looked-after children and when there is genuine interest in how best to help them, this book will be invaluable to all concerned – foster parents, social workers, teachers, psychotherapists and many others – in learning about what it really takes to listen to children.

Peter Wilson,
Young Minds

Acknowledgements

I owe a debt of gratitude to the children who appear directly or indirectly in these pages. In writing this book I used case notes of eighty children whom I met for individual therapy over the course of eighteen years. All had been referred to me by social workers, most were living in foster families and in residential homes. A few lived with their birth families or other relatives, whilst being on Child Protection Registers or having allocated social workers because there were Supervision or Care Orders in effect. A handful were adopted, with the adoptive placements being under great strain.

Thanks are due to very many people whose help and support I relied on: for reading chapters and being kind enough to not discourage me: Lesley Hollinshead, Tamsin Ford, Carol Hughes and Linda Dowdney. Peter Wilson managed to read the whole manuscript at a very rambling stage and still encouraged me. I owe the book's inception to my children, Seth and Natascha, for going abroad and leaving a gap that I had to fill. I owe the book's outline to Brigidin Gorman and Ian Butler of the Integrated Services Programme in Kent: they made me focus on essentials. My colleagues at ISP, at Heath Farm Family Services and at Brixton Child Guidance have all encouraged me. I did not help the children in these pages single handedly and in particular I relied on the work of Tamsin Ford, Janette Phillips, Rita Manfield, Chris Smith and Monica Lanyado.

I am grateful to Brigitte Josey who always believed I could write this. Thanks too to David Smallbone who directed me toward a publisher and then restrained from offering advice over a very lengthy period.

I write in longhand and Mandy Woodin produced the manuscript efficiently and cheerfully.

Finally, this book would be far less readable without the editorial help of Judith Edwards who read, advised and brought clarity to many of these pages.

*

Throughout the book, all names of persons referred to have been changed and every effort has been made to disguise their identity, but not in ways that change the meaning of the observation and clinical material.

Introduction

This book is written from the belief and with the experience that psychoanalytic child psychotherapy is a useful activity for multiply hurt and traumatised children. It can help them to heal and to trust again. Psychotherapy focuses on the obstacles to trust and the barriers to free communication, the obstacles and barriers that the self has raised to protect individuals from themselves and from others. These self-defences and the underlying anxieties which have called them into being, can be quietly and carefully given attention and can be understood by therapist and child. Losses can be mourned. Aggressions can be owned. The child can be helped to comprehend their feelings and their own responses. Gradually they can become 'master in their own house', aware of their own feelings and in charge of their own actions. Psychoanalysis, which traces back fears and anxieties to primitive states of mind and events long gone, requires each individual to own their own past and to take responsibility for their part in their own future.

However, psychoanalytic work with deeply mistrustful, traumatised children requires modification of therapeutic practice. The process has to be adapted to reach these otherwise unreachable children. Based on eighty experiences of therapy with children in care. I have written this book to demonstrate how therapy may be made viable. Because, in wanting to help children whose faith in adults is slim, whose experience of adults is dire and whose cynicism is often entrenched and well founded, therapists have to communicate in a way that might reach these individuals.

Principles and practices

(1) A sequestered space

Child psychotherapy is a process whereby a therapist meets regularly with a child once or more times every week, over a number of years. The setting of these meetings should be a neutral or special place, preferably one like a community mental health centre which the child will only visit for this purpose. This is preferable because of the powerful emotions released in therapy and the human facility for imbuing places and rooms with associations and feelings. Not just the encounter with the therapist but the building, the secretaries and the journey to and from therapy all tend to be felt as part of the process, particularly once therapy is really under way. Therapy attempted in a school setting, for example, has a more difficult mixture of connotations and meanings. When there is not much physical distance between therapy and the classroom there is greater likelihood that feelings spill over from one setting into another. An underlying principle of therapy is containment, the containment of hazardous and painful feelings within a safe, dedicated space and person.

(2) Time and other boundaries

Therapy lasts for a fixed and predictable amount of time, traditionally fifty minutes, called a 'therapy session'. Child psychotherapists are careful to begin on time and to end on time. They arrange sessions at the same time and on the same day or days each week. This care to keep to time boundaries functions as a clear division between the therapeutic encounter and other parts of life. Within the controlled setting of time and place, therapeutic rules of engagement are employed by the therapist.

Child psychotherapists generally see children in a dedicated, child-friendly room. The room will be equipped with sturdy, simple furniture, for example, a table and two chairs, some toy cupboards and, usually, a sink with running water. Some therapists have a good number of toys included in the setting: often a doll's house with furniture, soft toys and dolls, toy cars and a garage, a sand box and a water tray. Some therapists prefer a very uncluttered space where the child's individual box is the only selection of available toys.

In all cases, child psychotherapists take care that the room should not be full of other children's pictures and toys and that there are minimal 'don't touch' and 'no-go' areas. This is to communicate to the child that the empty space is for their exclusive use, free from the intrusions of others. As the therapy room is offered as a symbolic space for the child to make use of, care is taken to provide as neutral a setting as possible in order that it lend itself to the child's symbols and meanings. For, in this therapy room, at the child's therapy time, the child alone will be the sole focus of the therapist's interest.

(3) *A controlled setting*

Child psychotherapists do not allow interruptions – for phone calls or messages, for example – during the therapeutic session. Neither would a therapist leave the session, to fetch drawing paper or further equipment. The idea is that everything is arranged as far as possible to provide a special time apart from every day intrusions where the therapist and child can pay attention to the 'internal world' of the child.

(4) *The therapy box*

In order to facilitate the child's communications of their inner, psychological world, a box of small toys and art equipment is provided for each individual child. This box is for their sole use and is carefully stored between sessions – usually in a locked cupboard. The typical therapy box will contain a set of small family dolls (mother, father, children, grandparents all of the same ethnicity as the child's family), some toy domestic animal families (sheep, cows, pigs, horses), some fences or enclosures, some toy wild animals, some toy vehicles, plasticine, paints, coloured pencils, felt-tipped pens, a lead pencil, pencil sharpener, pencil rubber, string, glue, Sellotape and plenty of paper in a folder.

This box, presented to the child at each session in exactly the state it was left in the last session, performs a useful concrete link between therapy encounters. It comes to represent much of what transpires in therapy. For example, a child may well emblazon it with 'Keep out! For John and no one else' or decorate it with paint and drawings. The box may be orderly or messy, well or poorly used, a disintegrated mess of fragmented destroyed toys or full of creative constructed objects that are carefully tended.

(5) *Rules of engagement*

The child is given almost complete freedom over the use of the contents of the box as it is lent as a symbol of their inner world. Sad though it is to see a packet of pencils pummelled into dust and made useless for drawing, this is allowed in therapy. The therapist will address these actions as communications to her – perhaps of the child's inability to use hope and a need to quickly close down the possibility of creation, or to provoke anger and despair in her. More happily, the therapy box can become a container of the child's continuing ability to make good or to house rows of tenderly cared-for animals. Donna in Chapter 7 made a 'paper girl fed with paper' as an ongoing symbol of an impoverished needy self.

In therapy the child psychotherapist talks about the possible meaning of the child's actions and reflects aloud on these communications.

The encounter between therapist and child in a sequestered space, at predictable times and intervals and for an open-ended period of time, not usually less than once per week for a year, is the practical setting of child psychotherapy. Within that setting the therapist emotionally attunes herself to attend to the child.

Some key concepts of child psychotherapy

(1) Mental pain: anxiety

Sigmund Freud's founding of the process of psychoanalysis is well known and many of his insights have been incorporated into our culture and everyday understanding of each other. He demonstrated that underlying preoccupations and emotional impasses, the neuroses, were revealed when patients talked freely to an attentive therapist. Freud analysed the causes of mental pain, which he called **anxiety**. He outlined the **defences** used to keep painful thoughts away from the self. He thought that analysing these processes and **interpreting** them to the patient allowed them to gain insight into their feelings and to master them instead of denying and defending against these feelings. Freud pointed to the **transference** of feelings onto the therapist and the tendency to re-enact with the therapist earlier relationships that the patient has experienced. Crucially, transference of the first dependent relationship of infant to mother is projected onto the available therapist.

(2) Interpretation and containment

The concepts of **projection**, **transference**, **anxiety** and **defences** are still used today by psychoanalytically trained child psychotherapists.

However, as well as **interpretation** being a prime mechanism by which insight and change is encouraged, **containment** is now perceived as an equally important process. Melanie Klein, Wilfred Bion and others shifted the conceptual focus from one where problems were located in the internal psychological world to one where relationships between people were the core of difficulties. The confusingly named **object relations** theorists pointed to the inherently social framework of human feelings. The baby, who in anger feels like biting, bites a mother that he fears may bite him back. The earliest, most primitive feelings are nevertheless experienced as between the self and another. What is transferred therefore in a transference relationship is a two-person drama: both child and therapist are expected by the child to be playing reciprocal parts.

Taking in the child's projections, receiving them but not acting them out, is to emotionally contain the child's fears and fantasies. Containment, unlike interpretation, does not depend on intellectual understanding. It is an experience of being met emotionally that can be healing even without the child's intellectual understanding.

(3) The role of play

Whilst Sigmund Freud's patients used unguarded speech or '**free association**' as the vehicle by which their preoccupying thoughts would be revealed, Klein and Anna Freud pointed to the child's use of **play** as fulfilling the same function. Winnicott later expanded on the uses of play which occupies a between-world, between action and thought. In play children can concretely follow through a fantasised course of action, can act out their feelings and imagine the outcome, can experiment with different endings to inner dramas. Play therefore gives a window to the child's unconscious thoughts and feelings. Symbolic play is used by the therapist to understand the child's inner world. Interpretation can be made '**in the displacement**', for example, 'That monster chasing the little lamb seems to want to punish him for hitting the mummy sheep', or interpretation can link to an external situation, perhaps 'You expect a punishment for wanting to hit your mum this morning', or interpretation can be '**in the transference**': 'You think I may be like a monster and chase you for wanting to hit me'.

(4) Attunement and maternal reverie

Emotional attunement is the primary task of the therapist: what is called 'getting alongside' one's client. The therapist seeks to understand the child's world first from the child's point of view without censure or blame.

Close attention is paid to the young person in therapy. There is a focus on meaning, intent and the minutiae of what is emotionally exchanged between child and therapist. The therapist sets out to gather in and receive the emotional communications of the child. Using herself as a receptive feeling human being she enters into this unknown relationship with the child. Because human beings are empathic, reciprocal and able to feel and reflect on each other, a therapist is able to use herself as a barometer to gauge the child's emotional state. The process of being attended to, felt and thought about is in itself an emotionally containing experience. It has come to be thought of as one of the major curative actions of child psychotherapy. The often used prototype is that of infant with mother. The infant evacuates distress with which it cannot deal and is in a state of emotional pain. The mother in empathy takes in the infant's pain, sympathises and demonstrates to the child that she is aware of it, sharing the baby's distress. The mother copes with the pain, seeking relief for the baby, finding solutions to combat or cure pain. She offers comfort and the confidence that pain can be helped and borne. Bion (1971) called this 'maternal reverie', emphasising the essential elements of quiet, confident attentiveness of mother to infant.

(5) Psychoanalysed therapists

The most essential part of therapeutic equipment is the mind of the therapist. It is therefore of enormous importance that the therapist is self-aware and balanced in her dealings with clients. The strenuousness of the task, the critical nature of the therapist's own capacity and the necessity for her to distinguish her client's motives and feelings from her own is essential. Child psychotherapists have their own psychoanalysis over many years. We have a rigorous four-year postgraduate training. Supervision is essential for practitioners, no matter how experienced. Child psychotherapists register with a professional body which oversees an ethical code of practice and handles complaints and disciplinary procedures. Finally, child psychotherapists work as part of multi-disciplinary teams where they are constantly influenced by other professionals with alternative models of thinking and practice. Peer scrutiny and challenge go some way to providing a balance to the unequal power we have with our young clients.

(6) Classical child psychotherapy

Whilst there is really no classical analytic therapy as such, there are practices and techniques which have become commonplace amongst child psychotherapists. The training schools of child psychotherapy (see p. 182) are of course key players in institutionalising what was in Anna Freud and Melanie Klein's day a much more fluid practice. The necessity of teaching best practice has at times become an unthinking enactment of tradition. On the other hand it has fostered a disciplined, highly controlled service in a field that was open to amateurs. A fuller account of present practices in the field can be found in Lanyado and Horne, *The Handbook of Child and Adolescent Psychotherapy*, Routledge, London, 1999.

(i) The blank page

Child psychotherapists try to exclude their own personal business from therapy. Just as intrusions of phone calls and other people are kept away from the therapeutic hours, so the therapist keeps back her personal life and relationships to serve as a more facilitative 'transference object' (I am afraid we are stuck with the word 'object' for historical reasons. It's intended to mean 'the object of desire' rather than 'reification'). This means that there can be a certain lack of spontaneity in the therapist's demeanour and interaction with her client and their escort.

(ii) The controlled setting

The therapist tries to keep the boundaries of the therapeutic hour clear and this has also meant that what comes into the session and what is taken out is considered symbolically, and thus controlled. Children are usually discouraged from taking their paintings and creations out of the sessions. Three reasons are pertinent: one is that the symbolic meanings and transference value of the paintings becomes lost or difficult to follow. A second reason is that attention is taken away from the non-material gains in therapy. Thirdly, and most importantly, the containment and confidentiality of the session is breached by a stream of pictures being taken from the therapy.

(iii) Therapeutic neutrality

The child psychotherapist is at pains to allow hostile and negative transferences as well as positive transferences. Therefore the child is not to be jollied out of their hostility or seduced from their distrust. Rather these feelings are to be allowed, understood and interpreted. By bearing negative transferences with equanimity, the therapist allows the child to work through some of the more difficult aspects of earlier experiences.

A seminal paper by Anne Alvarez (1985) addressed the issue of analytic neutrality for 'borderline' psychotic children. She put forward the idea that what may seem neutral to one child may seem hostile to another. One may need to adjust one's 'neutrality' to adapt to particularly damaged children.

(iv) Confidentiality

A strict rule of confidentiality over sessional material was always promoted by child psychotherapists. The reasons for this were less often articulated but it was held to be part of the strict observation of boundaries: the therapist must not 'spill out' the child's feelings because she cannot contain them. The essence of therapeutic containment and reverie was thought to be breached if therapists shared their experiences of the child except in professional, controlled arenas, as in supervision. Also, following the model of adult psychoanalysis, it was assumed that children would not share their intimate feelings with therapists who would tell their secrets. It was assumed to be a betrayal of trust.

Adaptation of technique

The rules of classical technique sometimes need breaking for fostered children. My arguments for doing so and my belief in adapting child psychotherapy for the population of fostered children have been a major impetus in the writing of this book.

I have for the sake of brevity followed the convention which refers to psychotherapists throughout the text as female.

Chapter 1

Beginnings

First impressions

- what gets communicated
- the psychotherapeutic task
- debates about interpretation and the ego
- the use of psychotherapy as an assessment
- the importance of preventive work

Jenny, 9 years

'What's out there? Can we play outside? Why not? Whose is this? Does Mark O'Reilly come here? How does this work?'

She moved rapidly through my room, touching one toy after another, stopping at none of them, asking questions but giving little attention to my answers, bombarding me with dilemmas. When she came near me she rarely made eye contact and, as if on elastic, swiftly recoiled to the far walls, to the windows, to the door. At 9 years of age she was small and wiry, with an engaging but fleeting smile and boyish wavy fair hair. She smiled often and placatingly: it was a struggle to pause and resist her direct 'Can I? Why not?' Within minutes I felt unbalanced, slow, guilty at saying 'no' so often and with unclear reasons. With an effort I pointed out to her the cardboard storage box I had placed for her on the table. It was my standard issue for children in therapy: plain, larger than shoe-box size with a good lid and able to hold an array of stationery and art materials, Plasticine, some family dolls of a size that would fit the doll's house, some small toy farm and zoo animals with fences, a folder to keep any paintings and drawings in, a plastic container useful for finished Plasticine models and lots of paper. She looked at the box but did not approach it.

'What's in it?'

'You can look. It's for you to use.'

She turned back to an open box of Lego and began to rummage through it.

'Do you know how to make this?' she asked, pointing to an illustration on the box.

For a few moments we looked for pieces together and she tried to command me to make the construction for her. As suddenly as she'd come near to me she sprang away and, notwithstanding her dress, began to do handstands in the corner of the room, her legs perilously close to the windows. Her dress fell over her head, her knickers on view, her bare legs in the air.

'No, you make it, you do it,' she complained as I stopped the Lego building to watch her. I pointed out a better, safer section of wall for her to use, keeping a little distance from her, yet still, without warning, I found her legs catapulting into my arms. She wrenched herself free and, breathless and laughing, climbed up to the window and tried the catch which was fortunately securely locked . . .

In the fifty minutes we spent together on this first meeting alone (we had met days earlier with her social worker) she went several times up to the box that I had specified was 'for her'. Each time she seemed distracted by another idea, or played with something else; she never touched it or opened it. At our second meeting she seemed to ignore her box altogether and I again pointed it out to her. At our third meeting I noticed how she ricocheted from the box into swift breathless excitement. Or was I imagining it? Perhaps because the box had strong significance for me I was assuming, projecting onto her a reaction that was noteworthy. Perhaps lidded cardboard boxes are not particularly interesting. A stray wish for prettier plastic boxes that might be more attractive went through my mind. As she filled up the sink with water to see if a Lego construction would float I found a few unusual minutes of quiet to gather my thoughts. As she dashed away from the sink with a wet construction that she deposited back in the Lego box, I resisted the invitation to reprimand her and asked, 'Jenny, why do you never look in that box I've given you?' She went up to it then and touched the lid with both hands.

'What's in it?' she asked.

'Why don't you look and see? I replied.

'Has it got sweets in it? Chocolates?' she asked.

'What makes you think that?' I wondered aloud.

She moved away and to the window saying, 'If we had a skipping rope I can do a trick.' I didn't reply, allowing myself to continue being puzzled about the box. She looked directly at me then, from the safe vantage of several feet away.

'I bet you used to have chocolates in that box but probably they've gone now.'

'How would that be?'

'Probably the others have eaten them all by now.'

As the reader can see, there were many things going on in my encounter with Jenny: her wariness, her wish to control me, to keep me busy and at a safe distance, her wish to escape. I felt as if I were with a caged animal who was wary and predatory. But there was longing for contact here too: the sudden physical contact, the exposure of legs and knickers in excited energetic play, the bombardment of me into compliance, all added to my growing suspicion that she had been sexually abused. An aspect that I only noticed after the second and third sessions was that somehow pieces of Lego went missing from the room following her visits. So there was an undercurrent of trickery and distraction of me whilst she secretly took something from me. Did she think herself a thief, secretly enjoying the credulousness and carelessness of those with possessions? Or was she certain that she would never be given and would have to take, surviving on her wits as a scavenger, treasuring the detritus of adults the way street children pick up and appropriate effects in third world countries? The experience of being with her was one of struggle, unease, alarm. I felt her rapid changes of direction disconcerting. I was crowded by her rapid-fire questions and challenges. I seemed to have little room for thought, for feeling, for wondering, when I was with her. I was very puzzled and nonplussed by her. We met but we made little contact. We might have been sword-fighting or sparring. That was the emotional tenor of what was occurring.

But what comes back to me most clearly, is that sudden look, that moment of real contact when she said to me, 'I bet you used to have chocolates in that box but probably they've gone now.' She said this with an urgency and despair which were oddly at variance with the alluring idea of chocolates. At that moment what was conveyed to me was longing and sadness for what might have been, for what had been but had got lost. This communication was the crucial one in our encounter. Jenny, in three fifty-minute meetings, showed me what it is like to be anxious, mistrustful, ready to flee or fight, to be ever wary and ever on guard. But in a few seconds of real human contact she threw into me a kernel of sadness, of loss, of her attempt as a little girl to cover over her experience of an empty, depleted 'other', her experience of a gift that holds only disappointment.

Jenny caused me to wonder whether she was really impervious to the box I gave her or whether it was my own sensitivity to rejection that made me notice her lack of interest in the box. I had found myself wishing my gift was nicer, more attractive. Her later remarks showed me that I was not wrong to attribute this rejection to her, a transference of her own feelings from past disappointments to me and my gift. It was a counter-transference feeling that was aroused in me when I wished to improve my offering to a prettier plastic box. That is, it was a feeling aroused in my unconscious as a response to her unconscious communication.

If one imagines being Jenny's new foster mum, with subtlety and then more openly Jenny will give the message, 'You don't have what I need. I will not consider what you have on offer because I know it will disappoint and fail me.' The foster mother may have an equivalent thought to my wish for bright plastic: 'I don't have what this child needs: I wish I did. I'm not very good for her.' When these feelings are caught, traced back to their origins and considered consciously quite a different situation is the true one. This is a sad, disappointed and self-destructive child. She is robbing the potential mother. She is rejecting what is on offer without knowledge of what that is. A child who stays in this state is going to prevent good-enough mothering from reaching her. The beginning of therapy with Jenny then is to understand the communication of pain and disappointment with which she approached me. I need to feel it, to share it and to reach beyond my own vulnerable responses to it. I have gradually to absorb this knowledge into my perception of her and gently to disentangle it from the present on her behalf. So I will begin to draw these feelings to her attention, to notice them and name them. But more importantly, I will hold onto these feelings and not push them away, nor respond 'in the counter-transference' with either guilty placatory gifts or with retaliatory rejection. In the quiet of a therapy room, with time after and before each meeting, time in which to think and disentangle my responses, I can hope properly to understand our exchanges. This is the essence of psychotherapy. In effect I will, by example, feel and face the despair before we together relegate the pain to where it belongs – in the past.

In Kleinian theory (Klein 1975) one thinks of the unconscious encounter in therapy as one between child and mother. Or rather between the child and the child's idea of a mother – what is confusingly called 'the maternal object'. Object here refers to the 'object' of desire, meaning the target of the person's affections. Not every aspect of the meeting between child and therapist falls into this category, of course, but the therapist by her receptivity, by her restraint at performing other roles (not a teacher, not a friend, not a substitute real parent) hopes to filter and gather in those aspects of the child which are related to early assumptions about the mother. The situation of seclusion, of meeting one-to-one with a person whose task is to help with personal pain will automatically evoke some of these 'transferences'. Feelings experienced in bringing the earliest needs to another are bound to be awoken. The therapist scans through the mass of incident accumulating in the room and asks: 'What assumptions is this person making about me? What sort of "maternal object" am I for her?' It is therefore extremely important that the therapist keeps an open-minded stance toward the client and questions her own assumptions and projections. The therapist also tries to exclude her own actual and personal details from the sessions. Of course, the therapist is a particular human being with very many observable qualities that the client will correctly apprehend. But the more children are allowed to bring in preoccupations of their own, rather than those of the therapist, the more can be learnt. The more receptive the therapist, the more children will use assumptions and perceptions arising from their own personality and experiences. Accurate perceptions of the therapist show the child's intact receptivity. Inaccurate perceptions reveal unconscious aspects of the child and will become the material to be worked on. Children learn from their projections which are caught by the therapist and gradually reflected back to them. The child learns that unconscious ideas and past memories frame their own current experiences. Jenny, excited to be with me and to use me, cannot help but reveal her assumption that I must be tricked into providing for her. She is not simply open to what I can offer: she is in fact certain that I will disappoint her.

The first task of a therapist is to apprehend the children in all their communications, conscious and unconscious. So a therapist has to be aware of her own projections and distortions. We all see the world 'through a glass darkly' to some degree and indeed we have to have a personal framework on which to hang our experiences. But a therapist must strive for clarity between the emotional baggage that she herself brings into the room and that which belongs to the client. It is for this reason that psychoanalytic therapists have to have their own analysis as part of their training. We need to know what we project, where our common areas of confusion and distortion lie, where are our vulnerabilities and our strengths. We need to have scrutinised our own baggage so that we are more or less sure that the despair or anger or joy flooding the consulting room belongs to the client and not to ourselves.

Eloise, 16 years

A very angry, very powerful 16-year-old came to see me one day. She had been cajoled by her residential social worker to 'give me a try'. Her social worker thought I might help her through the maze of drinking bouts, drug overdoses, self-cutting, shoplifting and running-away episodes that had become her life. She was a tall, imposing girl with a pallor to her skin that made her look ill. Her hair was dyed black and cropped short and jagged. She looked hard, aggressive, fierce. Perhaps a warrior about to engage in battle might adopt this look: it said 'don't mess with me'. I felt intimidated by the way she swept into the room and sank into a chair, looking furious. The conversation we managed to have was fitful and awkward. She responded to my attempts to engage her with monosyllables and challenges. Eventually I had little choice but to say what seemed obvious: that she didn't want to be here and was annoyed that she had to talk to me. Instead of the angry response that I expected – in fact I was almost expecting a slap – she looked panic-stricken, fearful. I then realised how thin was her veneer of protective hostility and how much she feared this meeting. So I did my best to be non-threatening and matter-of-fact. I talked about therapy as a possible relationship where you can talk things over privately without repercussions. I said that I wouldn't be in the middle of her life participating in the plans about her placement (which she told me she hated), her education (she also hated that), her access to her boyfriend (a 30-year-old man), or her curfew (she was in a secure unit). I tried to explain that therapy is 'off to one side' as a place to talk and think. Of course, it depended on whether we two could get on together and, since we did not know one another, that was hard to predict. All I could do was offer to see her a few times and then she could tell me whether she thought it useful to continue or not.

In this way I tried to give Eloise control over the decision about therapy. I tried also to 'set out my stall' in a clear way: this is what is on offer. Perhaps, Eloise, you will, or perhaps you won't, find it useful.

By doing a lot of the talking at this first meeting I was, of course, missing what I could have been gathering in from Eloise. In an easier encounter I could let the young person set the agenda, I could sit back and let her preoccupations, her phrases, her expressions and emotions wash over me and filter away like a receding tide. I could be relatively passive, receptive and keep to the analytic stance, asking myself: 'What is this that I am being given? What sort of quality does it have? What is its meaning? How does she perceive me?' This is the process called 'gathering up the transference'. This was not possible with Eloise, however. She was scared of me and feared my perceptions: I guessed she wanted to give me nothing I could use to hurt her. In a younger child who is afraid it may be useful to offer back this insight in a gentle way: 'I think you might be afraid I'm like that monster in your game . . .', but sometimes this can be overwhelming if the fear is too acute. With a young woman of 16 years, there is the added difficulty of a loss of face, when to admit to fear or timidity cuts across the need to look poised and adult. So at the beginning it may be wiser for the therapist to act on the basis of her perceptions rather than interpret them in a classical analytic way.

Eloise was hostile and fearful. I tried to help her master these feelings, initially by demonstrating she had little to fear from me, later by reflecting back to her that I was unknown and she would have to experience our relating before she could judge whether it was like her fantasy of me or not.

In this way Eloise half-heartedly agreed to see me again. At our second meeting she was more poised and less afraid. After some brief pleasantries she launched into an account of sharing a room with a new resident at the secure unit. Eloise liked the idea of sharing because she did not much like sleeping alone. But this other girl wanted the light on and Eloise was not able to sleep with it on. It transpired that the light was a small night light and the other girl had agreed to have it as far away from Eloise as possible. But it was useless. For Eloise, just the knowledge that there was a light on in the room bothered her. On a rising note of indignation Eloise put to me this other girl's irritating habits and described the argument they had. She confronted me angrily: 'So who's right then, me or her?'

I re-described the situation she was putting before me as a dilemma that might apply to myself and herself. We were 'being told', or so it may seem to her, to share a therapy room. But she feared we were incompatible. I may want different things from her: she may find my wishing to throw light on things upsetting and irritating. But she wanted companionship, she didn't like being alone. The dilemma was so upsetting that she wanted an immediate end to it, a yes-or-no final solution. Yet, we could hear at the beginning of her account, a wish to share, a hope that she might not be alone in the dark.

Eloise regarded my interpretation with incredulity and then contempt. That's what she had heard about people like me, she replied. People like me twisted what was said and just went off onto something else. I did my best to assure her that I was not meaning to do this but that I did have a different way of thinking about these things.

However, this seemed all that was needed to intensify Eloise's anger. Her resentment at being made to come and her perception of the care staff and myself as self-seeking bullies and hypocrites came pouring out. There was a despair laced into her angry rejection of me which I could feel but could not address. An angry tidal wave seemed intent on buoying her up to the point where she was going to sweep out of the room. As she reached a sort of crescendo of anger and hostility about all adults, she gave me a sudden moment of sympathy and said, 'It's nothing personal. I never wanted to come.' I replied that she seemed to think this meant that we had to end, but it may be a good, honest place to begin. I saw the momentary hesitation as the idea reached her, but it was swiftly crushed. She was on her feet and out of the room, shouting for her escort to take her back in an angry and public display of her rejection of me.

The uncomfortable aftermath of this sort of encounter for the therapist is the question of whether my interpretation was precipitous and caused her rejection of me. The alternative, however, may be that one is bullied into compliance and collusion. In addition, holding back on honest exchanges can quickly make a therapy session feel boring to an ambivalent adolescent. Eloise found ambivalence an intolerable state. There was therefore little room for looking at opposing feelings or contradictory thoughts. She insisted on myself or the staff adjudicating between rights and wrongs, between herself and her roommate, between the part of herself that wanted to share and the part that was utterly intolerant of difference. Eloise sought to answer her dilemmas by powerful, final, precipitous action. This is anathema to therapy. Whether the small, overlooked wish to share and to not be alone in the dark was ever to be heard by her remained to be seen.

This illustrates one of the points on which theoretically Melanie Klein and Anna Freud diverged (Segal 1979: 42). Klein argued that unconscious fears are better brought out into the light where they will dwindle into more realistic proportions. Anna Freud was afraid of overwhelming the ego – the reality sense – by too great an acknowledgement of unconscious fantasy. Theoretically the two approaches are quite different and seem incompatible. Is the therapist to use her intervention to support and shore up a weak ego? Should some aspects of therapy be didactic, teaching the client what is real and well-founded, steering away from over-exposure to fantasy, feeling, imagination? Or is the therapist to assume a fearless exposing role toward fantasies, defrocking them of their powerful fantastical clothes? Is the therapist to name the feelings of dread which haunt the client? The theory concerns how ego-strength is built and the processes of development. Thus the argument between Klein and Anna Freud involved competing theories of infant development. Klein's theories emphasised the presence of reality sense in the infant from birth or before. She argued that the ego does not come into being through a process of construction – as, for example, Jean Piaget (1954) was to persuade us: reality built up by a process of investigation. In the Piagetian and Freudian child, reality-sense is won with difficulty and in the face of competing ideas. Klein, however, emphasised the child's cognitive integrity from early on, the child's perception of the world as accurate and acute but distorted through a veil of feelings, wishes, fantasies. For Klein, what stands in the way of a strong ego-sense is emotional distortion. Therefore she did not fear to damage the ego by focusing on these intervening fantasies.

Meanwhile, Anna Freud gave greater weight to developmental stage. She felt that young egos were bound to be weaker, more vulnerable. She emphasised therapeutic alliance, the therapist joining with the healthy part of the client before interpretative work could occur. For Klein this sometimes felt like collusion, like an inability to stand the negative transference which may come when clients identify the therapist with all the nasty ideas they have carefully locked away from the self. Anna Freud would perhaps counter that the negative transference will simply make clients more defended, more in the grip of defensive distortions in an attempt to protect themselves.

As a student I read these debates with enthusiasm and with awe. As a practitioner I know them as hugely over-simplistic attempts to push complex realities into a theoretical frame. Later theories stressed the notion of emotional containment, particularly following the writings of Wilfred Bion (1971: 72–82), the issues of when to 'hold onto' the client's feelings and when to give them back as interpretations became a larger, more complex, debate. There are many interesting contributions to this literature and the topic is now addressed with much greater subtlety and complexity (Sandler 1985: 3; Alvarez 1983).

Sitting opposite an angry and fraught 16-year-old Eloise I doubt that theoretical debates can be of immediate use. One has to make instant and largely instinctive decisions about how to answer and how to lead the conversation. Psychoanalytic theory and practice is an addition and a refinement to our communication skills: it does not replace ordinary communication. In ordinary discourse, we perceive and respond to each other with sympathy, with kindness. We also endeavour to balance our response to the situation of the other.

Vincent, 9 years old

Nine-year-old Vincent was living in a large, local authority community home when I met him. He had been pushed from pillar to post, from mother to father, to grandparents, to family friends, until his family one by one at this juncture in his life had abandoned him. He was a noisy, demonstrative, cheeky, streetwise lad who both exasperated and charmed those who knew him. In his meetings with me, however, he showed a heaviness, a despair that was heart-wrenching. He came into my therapy room with the weight of the world on his shoulders. It was only as I acknowledged and allowed this part of himself to be expressed that his considerable resourceful energy began to be released.

Our first meeting alone was characterised by Vincent's air of boredom. He had been playing outside on a slide until collected and brought in to see me. He seemed not to recall our introduction with his social worker the previous week until I re-described it to him. He seemed inured to the plans and explanations of adults and shrugged wearily but politely his acceptance of our arrangement to meet.

After a while he made quite a thorough exploration of the room, its toys and the box I gave him. Opening it, he was impressed that the handful of things I had presented to him were new. 'Are these new paints then?' and 'Is this mine now?' were two poignant themes. He gradually settled to a very skilled model-making of a slide and a swing. I said that he was bringing into the room what he had wanted to do and missed out on outside. He laughed at this and quickly included me in his play so that we were soon sharing the mini-playground he had made. He kept lapsing into inactivity. The room was heavy with the effort he seemed to make to shake off a strong sense of weary despair. The Plasticine stuck to the table and he tore it off anxiously, worried that it had made marks, excusing himself and apologising resignedly. I made clear that he was allowed to make some mess in here. We were hoping to deal with some very messy feelings so that therapy was a good place for messes. He took this in swiftly and shrewdly. He made toy cars skid, swerve and crash dangerously. Then he played an elaborate game of a rubbish van carefully collecting, transporting and tipping rubbish into the dump. The rubbish pile was put neatly before me, on the table where I had said messes were allowed. When we got to the end of our time he swiftly put each piece into his box. 'I want to come tomorrow. It's nice here isn't it?'

Some young people like Vincent have an instinct for and acceptance of the symbolic nature of play. Of course, there was also Vincent's hunger for relationship and his considerable experience and skill at new encounters. He had learned well how to draw people to him. His despair was felt in his anxiety that relationships quickly sour, get messed up and result in rejection. Vincent was initially tired at the idea of another relationship. He then became hopeful that it could be new, his own. He panicked at the assumption that a mess would be made and I would be intolerant of it. Then he seemed to have some hope that we could deal with unwanted 'rubbish' between us.

By our third meeting I had already made clear that Vincent could continue in therapy with me. However, we faced a break during the six-week summer holidays so that the assessment reports could be written and practical plans for his therapy finalised. He was in transition, probably resident for one year in his current placement whilst plans for permanency were sorted out. For this needy boy the hiatus was fraught. He viewed with open suspicion the plan that we would meet again after the summer holidays. His fear was that it would go wrong. He spent time making a round Plasticine circle in which he eventually placed a tiny figure of a boy. Then forty minutes was given over to a loud and exciting game where emergency vehicles, ambulance, police cars and fire engines had races to see who was the best. At the end of the session as I helped put these away I asked, 'What is this circle?' He replied, 'Oh it's a hole. He's fallen down there . . . we'll get him out next time . . . maybe.'

Jake, 7 years, and Philip, 5 years

Some children are referred to me without the intention for long-term therapy. A few exploratory meetings can be used to help define the child's internal situation and to give to the social-work team and to the child themselves some thoughtful reflections on their needs. This sort of assessment can be useful to everyone as long as the rules of engagement are clear. In assessment work I apply very different rules of confidentiality. I make clear to the young person that my meetings with them will be reported back to the social worker, the foster carer, the parents and perhaps the court. Of course, this limits what children may tell me during these meetings. Despite this, many children use these sessions to explore their current concerns and they often use our few meetings reflectively.

It has struck me over the years how useful such an emotional snapshot can be for social-work teams trying to fit services to the needs of accommodated children. Social workers have insufficient time or permission to get to know the child themselves. In addition, psychoanalytic emphasis on internal identifications and the importance of emotional processes prove to be stable indicators of a child's psychological traits.

In this style of work I have often seen siblings who are temporarily in foster care whilst various assessments are completed. For example, two brothers, Jake and Philip, were referred to me to assess their future suitability for psychotherapy and for an assessment of their emotional needs. Residential staff of the unit where they were temporarily accommodated, stressed the difficulties that Jake, the 7-year-old brother, presented. He was moody and demanding, he was emotional and often cried, sometimes he begged to be allowed to stay away from school as he was too upset to attend. By contrast no one was as concerned by

5-year-old Philip. He was cheerful and combative. Although he got into fights and arguments, the staff saw him as a survivor who got by without too much fuss. Both boys had been physically badly assaulted by their mother's boyfriend. The extent and frequency of their injuries and their mother's refusal to leave this violent partner indicated that they would not be returning to her care. The long-term plan was for their permanent placement in foster care.

Jake presented very much as the staff had described, as a boy who wore his heart on his sleeve. He told me about his hatred of 'Uncle Bill' and then gradually and hesitatingly of his love for his mother. He was in effect in a state of mourning that he had to leave her. His relief at my understanding and receiving his grief was palpable. He came readily to our few sessions and wanted to meet me as many times as he was allowed, despite his temporary situation. He used his sessions to good effect, gathering up his memories, good and bad, about his mother and trying to come to terms with her abandonment of him. He was understandably concerned about his future and drew a picture of a boat in the middle of a very choppy sea. He told me that it had slipped its anchor and that it did not know where it would end up. Despite the painfulness of being with him I was impressed by Jake's struggles to come to terms with his situation. He used the help he was given and he was sound enough to ask for more. He was clearly fond of his brother and his relationship with friends was good. A trusting kernel of himself seemed to have survived the abusive episodes of assault although I was told that he remained extremely wary of men.

By contrast, my heart sank after meeting Philip. It was true that Philip was tougher, less collapsed than Jake, but this was largely because he was in a state of identification with his abusive 'uncle'. His games were full of sadism and violence. His rivalry with the other children that I saw drove him to lay traps in my room for them. In the several sessions when we met I saw no indication of empathy, of kindness, of much tender feeling at all. His activities in the room concerned bullying and controlling me. When I intervened he interpreted this as my bullying superiority over him. I was extremely alarmed by his presentation and strongly recommended that he receive remedial therapeutic help as soon as possible.

In the event, both boys went to a long-term foster placement and, when this broke down two years later, to a residential facility. Many years later I came across Philip who sadly had been a frequent client of the Juvenile Justice System and spent some of his teenage years in secure accommodation. By contrast, his brother Jake had managed to steer clear of the worst of these difficulties and was maintained in foster care.

Anecdotal as this story is, I do think that psychoanalytic assessment of emotional state and recognition of characteristic defences provides a reliable guide to a child's needs and adjustment. Personality traits are likely to be enduring. The pity of this story is the failure of provision where specialist help for Philip was so clearly indicated. The assumption that psychotherapy is expensive and an optional extra for a child like Philip is ridiculous when contrasted with the cost of his career as a young and increasingly dangerous criminal. At 5 years of age one could have had some hope of diverting him from this course.

Chapter 2

A view from the bridge

Children in transition

- – external and internal worlds
- – the value of professional alliance
- – deficiencies in practice
- – networking
- – treatment length
- – multiple points of view
- – when therapy is not necessary

Children come to therapy through adults. It is because adults are worried about a child and have hopes that therapy can help that child and therapist ever meet. The views and understandings of the adults therefore are of critical importance to child therapy for, even where a young person asks to see a therapist, or wants someone to talk to, it is adults who arrange, who decide, who say 'yes' or 'no' to the endeavour. The child, the parents and the therapist will all have their own ideas about therapy and, to a greater or lesser extent, their own agendas. The situation then, when a child's care is shared between local authority social services and parents, brings yet more adults and more agendas into the picture. Routinely this will add the social worker, the team manager and budget holder and the foster parents or residential workers. All of these adults will need to agree to a working contract, initially for assessment and then for treatment if this is indicated.

In the eye of the storm, as it often seems, there is a child whose distress needs to be considered from his or her own individual viewpoint. This is the '*sine qua non*', the 'without which nothing is worth doing' of therapy. A therapist must not allow the social workers' conviction or a parent's preoccupations or a foster carer's despair or a social work department's panic to obscure the child's point of view. A child and adolescent psychotherapist will therefore have to try to absorb the concerns of all these different parties, to hear their distress and try to contain it whilst leaving her emotional intelligence as unbiased as possible for the communications of the child.

Who needs therapy?

Children defined as 'in need' by social workers are not necessarily children in need of psychotherapy. It is plain, however, that a large proportion of children who have to live separately from their parents and who become looked after in residential settings or in foster families are often emotionally needy as well. Many of these children will be multiply traumatised and will have suffered neglect or abuse. Some children will respond with emotional turmoil, feeling depressed and dejected, whilst others are moody, angry and prone to outbursts of temper. Children can, of course, move on from these states, begin to steady themselves, accept help and adapt to better conditions.

Some children, however, become stuck. When I think of what characterises children in need of therapy I think of those who have become stranded behind defences that they once needed but which are now an obstacle to their moving on. Philip (see Chapter 1), who identified with a sadistic bully, may have thereby saved himself from terror when he lived with 'Uncle Bill'. But Philip in the community residential home is a sadistic bully of other terrified children. Philip in school is a cynical boy who trusts no one and will not let down his guard to learn anything. Philip's assumption that other people must be manipulated into providing for him is a boy on a path to criminality.

Social workers often refer children for therapy in the midst of catastrophic change and upheaval. When an abused child is placed away from home it is understandable and appropriate that help is sought for their emotional well-being. However, a bewildered child having to get used to a new family, a new school and the experience of separation from all that is familiar may not welcome nor be able to make use of yet another professional stranger, a therapist. Therapists have therefore traditionally exercised caution in seeing or treating these children (Boston and Szur 1983: xiii). Such children are often in transition whilst their long-term care is being planned or evolving in the light of events. It makes little sense for a therapist to be presented as an emotional anchor in the chaos if it is unclear for how long the child is likely to be able to attend therapy sessions.

It is as well to assess whether the child's capacity for adaptation and change, their ability to use foster care and social-work support is all that is needed. The message to a child that their grief or distress can only be received by a psychotherapist may be unhelpful. It can be a message of rejection to a hurting child: 'I cannot bear to listen so I'll send you to a professional.' Would any of us feel comforted by such a response to our distress? But if the child is being listened to and nothing seems to help or they need something more, then therapy can be considered.

Assessment of a child's emotional needs and a few exploratory meetings with a therapist can be useful even in the midst of uncertainty. I have met many children and young people in these conditions and the meeting can furnish beneficial insights into the child's state for both carers and the child him- or herself. Short-term work and crisis interventions may also appear as a possibility once one has met the child. I have sometimes been persuaded by assertive social workers to meet children when I judged it unlikely to be helpful. Then I have found that the social worker was right: this particular child's needs outweigh the cautions of timing and planning and I have been glad to continue seeing my young client even as we wait for the court to decide on Care Orders and related issues.

Perhaps the most useful piece of advice for therapists and social workers considering therapy for children in transition is that we are not knowledgeable enough to make hard and fast rules. Instead of telling ourselves that we should not treat children in short-term temporary placements as I did (Hunter 1993a), we should simply voice openly to carers and child alike, the uncertainty and hazards of these meetings. We need to judge our interventions on a case-by-case basis.

Child psychotherapists working with children under the protection of Care Orders have to acquaint themselves with the 1989 Children Act, the framework of partnership with parents and the idea that several people will share the right to give permission and receive feedback on a child's assessment and progress in therapy (Butler and Roberts 1997). The sheer number of adults involved and the difficulties of liaison make these cases time-consuming and complex to manage. They also represent a daunting amount of emotional work for a single therapist. Traditionally in Child Guidance Clinics these cases were held by two colleagues, one of whom would see the child individually, the other of whom would network the case. I have found that it can also work well where the allocated field social worker and therapist form a good alliance. The social worker concentrates on external and practical issues and I concentrate on internal and emotional issues. However, any psychotherapist working with a looked-after child will find it necessary to keep abreast of the external practical events of the child's life as well and to attend case reviews and planning meetings as a matter of course. I learnt this lesson the hard way when I failed to realise the importance of one child's care plan.

The child's Care Plan and the network

Jenny (in Chapter 1), had been referred to me for assessment for ongoing therapy. Because it was clear to me that she was in need of therapy I was glad to agree with the referring social worker that I see her regularly. I set up therapy within the residential home and advised that I see her three times a week for a minimum of a year. Whilst it was planned that she be placed for eventual adoption the social work department's view was that she was unlikely to be placed in less than a year and this was partly my reason for treating her so intensively. However, three months into her therapy an offer to foster her with a view to adoption was received. In the event she was moved six weeks after I first heard about this. The family-finding workers were not aware that in therapy I was at pains to encourage trust and dependence in this fiercely wary child. I had not attended her reviews and planning meetings because I was fearful of losing my concentration on her 'internal world' and stepping too far out of my therapist's role. I had not even warned Jenny that I may be an unreliable source of help for her. Belatedly attending her case review I could not oppose the plan to move her as my colleagues made clear how few chances for adoption she would have, a child of 9 years, with her level of difficulty. It was a painful lesson for me because I saw that, despite my meaning well, my practice was deficient.

Of course, there are few certainties in life and such disruption could occur without contributory negligence from anyone. But I have since taken care to talk openly to the child about the limits of my commitment and the child's situation. I have also emphasised to the social-work team the nature of the slow, intense, reliable, consistent framework of psychotherapy and the danger of adding to the losses and abrupt discontinuities in these children's lives.

Therapists need to know and keep abreast of the long-term plans for an accommodated child. Long-term therapy needs to be included in the care plan. Changes of social worker or funding or placement breakdowns will all have implications for the relationship between child and therapist. Therapists also need to keep abreast of current developments in the child's life. Unlike work with children in their parents' sole care, responsibility and knowledge about looked-after children's lives are often spread between several people who may not coordinate well. Psychotherapists must take their place in these networks and play their part in keeping the child in mind.

Despite the disruption to Jenny's therapy, my experience has been that many children placed in 'short-term' or 'temporary' placements can use therapy effectively and not necessarily for just a short time. Of twenty children that I treated in temporary care I calculated the average length of their therapy was 1 year 10 months per child (Hunter 1993a: 218). During the same ten-year period the average length of therapy for children whose placement was described as 'permanent' or 'long-term' was 2 years 4 months. Effective networking and communication between professionals is probably the factor that contributes most to successful maintenance of a child's therapy. Therefore I have found it possible to sustain a relationship with the most difficult to engage children who perceive very astutely that the adults are committed to their attendance.

Different points of view

When a child is referred for psychotherapy and they are looked after by local authority social services the therapist needs to find out and hold onto a great deal of information, factual as well as emotional. Piecing together a child's life story and trying to identify gaps and omissions takes considerable work. I have rarely to receive a referral that does not require asking further, usually basic questions such as what incident was it that brought this child into foster care or what is the nature of mother's illness or is that child's father the same as this child's? In other words, basic factual information is often not presented and needs to be requested. Detective work and patience are therefore useful attributes during referrals.

Because children in public care often lead shattered, discontinuous lives, information about them becomes fragmented and lost. Their sense of themselves and their worth is harder to maintain if no one can even remember, for instance, that they lived with Nan in Southampton before she died. These children lack the sense that people know them, know about them in the ordinary continuous way that children in their own birth families take for granted. If a therapist is hoping to know a child intimately and unconsciously, they can at least take care to absorb these facts of the child's life.

It is also the case that in long-term therapy of three or four years the therapist can become the person who has known this child longest. Therapists of looked-after children have extra responsibility for gathering up and integrating the child's experiences. For some children this aspect of therapy alone is a valuable therapeutic experience: being remembered, being known, being important.

Natalie, 12 years

Natalie at age 12 was referred by her social worker for individual therapy, largely at her foster mother's request. Natalie was becoming difficult, stubborn and disobedient. She did not listen or seemed to forget what she was asked to do. When I requested information from her social worker it was evident that he was new to her case and found the three-volume case records somewhat difficult to master. I agreed to go to the social work offices and read the files, collecting for myself the information I found useful. Much of it was only indirectly connected with Natalie as she was a child from a family of many children all of whom had been in and out of care.

Natalie's history

Natalie's birth mother was portrayed as an intellectually limited, friendly, slovenly, boundary-less woman. She had many boyfriends, was perpetually 'engaged' and had married twice. The children were from three different fathers. All of Natalie's older half-siblings were accommodated outside the family by the time she was 3 years old but her mother fought fiercely to retain the care of Natalie, the youngest. Natalie was called 'baby' by all her birth family all through her life with them.

All of Natalie's older brothers and sisters had been sexually abused by various boyfriends of mother's. The children had, over time, been removed one by one but had continued to visit and drift in and out of mother's home. It seemed that there was sympathy for this hapless mother who neglected, could not protect, but seemed fond of her children. In Natalie's case she had been finally removed after several short episodes in foster care, when she had been discovered once again as a 3-year-old, filthy and with infected nappy sores, tied into her pram. Placed with a long-term foster family she gradually seemed to catch up on walking and talking and by the time she was 6 she was assessed as 'low average' compared with her peers.

Natalie had improved greatly with her foster parents' care. Despite doubts about her intellectual capability she was maintained in mainstream school with extra help. Now she was 12 her foster parents noticed how little she could sustain relationships with friends, how immature and unfocused she continued to be and, in their words, 'that she seemed to be falling back, not growing up like other girls'. A drifty, dreamy girl with an odd gait and body posture, Natalie seemed to ignore encouragement to be more mature and clung to her babyish status. She was terrified of her birth mother who had twice-yearly contact. The visits were preceded by Natalie's loss of bowel control and sleepless nights. 'Don't let me go back to that witch,' she begged her foster carers. During contact with her mother Natalie was showered with babyish presents. Later she became surly and argumentative with her foster carers, picking quarrels over nothing.

The foster carers' point of view

Mr and Mrs Langton were deeply attached to this child and Mrs Langton in particular had invested a remarkable amount of time and energy in helping Natalie. She had devotedly restored Natalie's failing health by discovering the child's allergies to certain foodstuffs and she had pursued cosmetic surgery for the girl. She had taught Natalie to read and to play the piano. In fact, Natalie had shown good musical ability and Mr Langton, a pianist himself, had encouraged her with lessons and rewards so that Natalie was a more than competent pianist. She could not master reading music, however, and this limited her success at formal examinations. It was evident that Mr and Mrs Langton had determined to compensate for and heal Natalie's poor start in life.

Despite both foster carers' pride in Natalie, a certain amount of weariness crept in to their descriptions of her. I thought that their implicit request of me was that I should succeed where they had failed. I should make her into the normal 16-year-old they hoped she would one day be. For what would become of Natalie, and how would it feel for them if after all these efforts she was not right, not properly mature?

The social worker's point of view

Because Natalie's care was competently managed by her foster carers the former social worker who had been allocated to her seemed to have had minimal contact with her. Anyway, Natalie was not overly fond of social work contact as she had in the last few years disliked feeling different from her older sister, the natural daughter of the Langtons. In some ways the social workers had had more to do with the natural mother who was often demanding further contact with the reluctant Natalie.

This newly appointed social worker confided to me that he questioned the access of Natalie's mother to her. For whose benefit was it, he wondered: Natalie's or her mother's? I supported this re-examination of the care plan. It was apparent to me that Natalie's foster carers had thought about adopting her but lacked the income to give her all the extra things like piano tuition that they felt she needed. They had been told that Natalie needed access to her mother, and against their better judgement they had felt they could do nothing but comply.

Eventually this social worker helped the Langtons adopt Natalie (with an allowance) and this delighted her and relieved them. She seemed not to feel ambivalent over her mother but maintained her angry dismissal of her. The birth mother, despite her protests, seemed to relinquish Natalie fairly easily. She had been fond of Natalie's former social worker and there was some evidence that she missed the visits more on that account. The foster carers claimed that Natalie's mother often ignored Natalie in favour of any other adult who was present.

Referral for therapy therefore occurred at the same time as re-examination of Natalie's care and an eventual shift to a more appropriate permanency in her life. Whilst these developments were yet to occur, however, I agreed to assess Natalie with a view to therapy.

The child's point of view

Natalie came willingly to see me and was pleased that I had a doll's house and a room full of toys. She presented as a much younger child than 12 years but with an emotional frankness that was endearing. I noticed that in one of the games she played a girl who was run over by a car. An ambulance came along, picked up the girl and took her to hospital. The car driver was taken to the police station, shouted at for 'being careless' and locked in prison. I made the comment that the girl had been helped, and that this happened before the bad driver was punished. Which was more important? 'You mustn't leave her there bleeding!' she answered me indignantly. To Natalie it was obvious that help must come before vengeance. I reflected that not every child that I see is as sound.

On our second meeting Natalie lined up the animals and with slow, sleepy patience tried to arrange them nose to tail in a long line. There was something sensual, perhaps sexual in her careful positioning of them. She looked at them, readjusted them, looked at them. The looking seemed to be an activity for her, soporific, soothing. She began to suck her thumb and look at me. Her eyes glazed as she rhythmically sucked her thumb and gazed and gazed at me. Whatever I said to her she seemed to ignore and then to my surprise she came up close and began to stroke my arm, my face, my hair. I moved away but had to stop her quite firmly from continuing. I had an odd feeling that she was trying to merge with me, climb in through my eyes, immerse me with her in her sleepy world.

On our third meeting I talked this over with her. She smiled sweetly and blinked longingly at me. 'You're my friend,' she said, again coming close and wanting to touch my hair. Again I had to be very firm to stop her, whilst she merely stopped rather than took in my discomfort.

Being with Natalie was an experience of drifting out to sea in a horizonless empty space. Lulling us along with her rhythmic thumb-sucking or quiet stroking, Natalie seemed to receive a primitive pleasure in looking, in feeling, that bypassed the need for communication, for difference, for noticing that I was someone she did not really know.

I thought of her being tied into her pram, watching the activities in her family. Her preoccupied neglectful mother had rarely picked her up, fed her, changed her. Had Natalie adapted herself by self-soothing stroking and the fantasy of merger, of drift and dream and latching on with her eyes, far away from the painful and uncomfortable sores on her bottom?

I interrupted Natalie's reveries as best I could. Instinctively I felt that I could never gain her attention by 'drifting out to sea' alongside her. So I asked lively practical questions about her life at home, at school, with birth mum. She talked about her birth family with vehement disgust and told me that she wanted to stay always with mum and dad Langton. She liked school, but only the teachers – the girls made fun of her. She sighed and looked for the first time distressed. She spoke warmly of her foster sister. She spoke proudly of her piano playing. She told me that she was going to watch her dad play at a concert next week. The soporific mood dispelled and she seemed again an immature but ordinary girl who was not very happy at school.

The school's point of view

It is often useful during an assessment to see children in their school setting amongst their peers and to gather reports and observations from their teachers. This practice has implications for the transference relationship which may be disturbed by the therapist's appearing in the school setting. I would therefore not conduct such a visit when regular therapy has started. As a part of the assessment process, however, I do find that it demonstrates to children the therapist's attempt to bring together the whole of their lives within the net of understanding. The practice mitigates against unhelpful splits in the child's behaviour. Children soon learn that therapy is different from the assessment process. I went to visit Natalie at school. Natalie's teachers welcomed my enquiries because they were quite concerned about her. In the classroom Natalie could not really keep up with the general activities and was given simpler versions of the work of the others. The other girls were, in my observation, quite kind to her but, during play time, she drifted off alone, seeming to isolate herself. This was possibly as a result of earlier rejections by her classmates.

Her class teacher felt that Natalie was misplaced in this mainstream school and that Natalie was often in a world of her own.

The therapist's point of view

Therapy is about enabling emotional and psychological changes in a person. Therapy cannot resolve access visits that re-traumatise a child who remembers her mother with fear and anxiety. Therapy cannot make happy a child who is placed in the wrong school. Or fulfil for well-meaning, admirable foster parents, their wish to have their child reach their too high expectations.

Therapists therefore have to carefully assess what they are being requested to do and decide whether it is viable.

I spoke tactfully but frankly with Mr and Mrs Langton together with the social worker. I raised the questions that had been raised for me and gave them time to consider and discuss these concerns. I let them know that I thought Natalie had some strange behaviours that I guessed were adaptations to her past. But I was worried that her school life might be too difficult and cause her to rely on fantasy and isolation as she had done long ago. Would a 'special school' placement furnish her with a level of work she could comprehend whilst giving her peers who were more on a par with her? Were we now doing her a disservice by expecting too much of a child who had very nice attributes but was intellectually limited?

In the event Mr and Mrs Langton found their own solutions to Natalie's school and peer difficulties. They sought out friends for her outside of school at clubs and musical activities. They helped her join the school choir and an out-of-school orchestra.

Natalie came to therapy with me for a year and gained very limited insight into her dreamy defences. And Mr and Mrs Langton, whom I also saw regularly, gradually adjusted their sights to realise that Natalie's very real good qualities would not disappear just because she was learning-disabled. Natalie matured into an adult who would always need added protection in life. But she held down a job, she managed semi-independence within her parents' home and she continued to love playing the piano.

The birth parents' point of view

In Natalie's case it did not seem helpful for me to interview her birth mother so I relied on information gained by my social work colleague. Yet in other cases it can be very useful to gather an early history of the child from the mother and at the same time absorb impressions about the mother's relationship to the child. Fathers are rarely available in the population of children I see, but of course the same is true of them. I have found too that looked-after children really appreciate the fact that I have taken care to find out as much as possible about them. Even when a parent is negative or hostile, children seem to find the fact that I have met with their parent an important and significant event. Twelve-year-old Jeremy, for example, referred by his social worker because he was scapegoated at home, was diffident about my involvement. Then I met Jeremy's mother and found that she wanted me to see if he was 'schizophrenic'. Jeremy was certainly nothing of the kind. He was a boy who felt rejected by his mother's disappearance from his life in his early years. Mother herself had suffered from depression and when she came back to her children after an absence of some years she expected that they would understand her needs and settle down in her care. Jeremy, desperate to reunite with the mother he missed, vented his anger and rage on his siblings and eventually came into foster care. He was quite unmanageable at school and was permanently excluded. Anxious to protect the poor attachment his mother had for him, Jeremy idealised and agreed with his mother. His anger and disappointment sought other outlets.

Jeremy's mother made clear that, since I did not agree that her son was mentally ill, it was a waste of time my seeing him. Reluctantly, however, she agreed not to oppose his treatment.

Jeremy was relieved that I still wanted to see him after his mother had told me 'how bad he really is'. He came without fail and used his sessions well. I was far more appreciative of his situation, having met his mother. I realised that his diffidence to me was partly out of loyalty to his mother. We had to have a relationship that realised his awkward situation and where I had to find a way to deal with his mother's negativity toward him without making it worse. As this was one of the major tasks Jeremy himself had to resolve it was crucial that I join him in this. In addition, had I not seen his mother I would not have fully understood Jeremy's occasional reference to 'being psycho' and his fear of it.

The foster family's points of view

Working with children in their birth families, most initial consultations involve meeting the child with their whole family. Seeing a child with mum and dad, with brothers and sisters, gives the therapist a valuable view of the family's interactions and the referred child's place in their family. It also gives an idea of what individual therapy for one child may mean to other family members.

Children in a foster family can rarely be seen in this context and the loss of this vision for the therapist is considerable. Should one try to see the child with the members of his current home? Sadly this is generally impractical. A foster family may object to bringing their birth and fostered children to a meeting of one child's therapist. In the specialist foster-care provisions in which I have worked, so many of the children are in therapy that a continual round of meeting each child's therapists would be the result. Fostered children are often moving on, new additions arrive and the 'family snapshot' that one may have taken at the beginning will no longer fit six months down the road. This in itself is instructive, of course: it should bring to our attention how shifting and changeable is the life of a looked-after child.

It may be coincidence but in the few instances where I have been privileged to meet a child's foster family the most striking impression to me has been the burden placed on the natural children of the family. Perhaps the cases I have seen have been biased by a difference in the degree of protection afforded the natural children evidenced by bringing them to meet me. Perhaps the natural children in these instances have been glad of the opportunity to meet someone to whom they can pass on the difficulties of living with a particularly difficult fostered child.

I think of a likeable and articulate 14-year-old natural daughter, Tamsin, who was living with a furiously angry and destructive fostered 10-year-old who wrecked her possessions and used language which shocked and embarrassed her. A year after the end of the fostered girl's two-year therapy with me, Tamsin contacted me. She wanted to share her alarm that this 'monstrous' sibling was being fully adopted by her parents. There was a tone of 'this is your fault' about the contact which persuaded me that I should respond. I hoped that I was not breaking too many boundaries to see her. Her parents agreed to this course of action and to its confidentiality. On our two meetings she made very clear her grief over the loss of a peaceful and innocent family life before the 'importing' of disturbed behaviour into her home. She had been shocked and distressed by details of abuse that her foster sister imparted to her.

She was also upset by her own failure to be tolerant. Hearing her out, I helped her disentangle the fact that she had a right to guard her own territory and possessions. I identified for her the sense of guilt that she felt at not being a parent or a therapist to her foster sister. It was this guilt that she was fending off with displays of anger. This interpretation seemed to bring her great relief. I felt keenly how preoccupied the adults were with fostered children and how neglected a birth child may feel, implicitly expected to act like a foster parent herself. It was interesting that she chose to give this anguish to me, her sister's therapist. This was not mainly, I believe, that she wished to spoil the sister's therapy. It was because she needed to juxtapose the part of herself identified with a therapeutic response to her sister with an angry, resentful part of her, robbed of the peaceful childhood she felt she should have had. By seeing her, I legitimised her own needs. She went away considering whether in the longer term she might have therapy for herself.

This and other experiences have increased my respect for foster families and made me more careful to not add to their burdens. Meeting foster parents I am at pains to hear their experience of the fostered child and to be supportive of their efforts. Foster parents may have had no experience of therapy or they may have their own attitudes toward it. I think with shame of the carelessness with which some professionals, child psychotherapists included, treat these parents. They are not powerful in the decision-making over children. Their employment status with a local authority is telling: they have no employee rights, no pension, no sickness benefits, little protection, variable training, variable support. If a child assaults them, alleges abuse, wrecks their property, they usually carry the brunt of the harm for months without redress. Angry, disempowered birth parents, scapegoated and abused youngsters may recognise in foster carers a place to dump the blame of which they want to be rid. Well-protected professionals may unwittingly join in. There is then plenty of room for misunderstanding and room for conflict of interests between foster carers and therapists.

Some foster carers are easily threatened by psychotherapists. They may feel that they are being pushed aside or that their handling of a child is under scrutiny or criticism. They may be unwilling participants in a referral made by the social work team which will involve them in awkward journeys for appointments but little else. Worse, they may have their own need to be the child's sole rescuer and deeply resent the intrusion of a psychotherapist in this relationship. Child psychotherapists will have had their own rescue fantasies well analysed, and we hopefully have some insight and control over our own illusions of grandeur. Foster carers with scant training will often have to rely on their natural capacities of goodwill and generosity and on their natural self-defences and insight. They are on the receiving end of painful projections, exhausting behaviour, rejection, bad temper, hostility and abuse from fostered children, and their defences may be needed.

It is of the utmost importance to psychotherapy with a fostered child that the attitude and opinion of the foster carers are taken into account by the therapist. In the best work, child psychotherapist and foster carers make a mutually supportive alliance. They usually both experience at first hand the child's difficult behaviour. They need to avoid being split into 'good therapist' and 'bad foster mother' or vice versa, and to understand this if it happens. They need to respect confidentiality as freeing the foster parent of concerns over therapy material and not as a function of a power relationship between them as competitors. They need to be perceived by the child as cooperative, working together and not mutually critical. These children have often come from emotional war zones where adults gave free rein to hostility and vendetta. Psychotherapy, which takes place in a setting of mutual discord or distrust between therapist and carers, will do more harm than good if it replicates these civil wars.

I believe good practice demands that the child's therapist and the foster carers should meet once every term, that is minimally three times a year, and should keep in unobtrusive contact as the need arises. A child needs to know that the adults work together behind the scenes: they do not need to feel that every time a pebble is dropped in a pond at home the ripples reach the therapy room. One of the most valuable aspects of therapy, of course, is that there should be no repercussions from therapy back into a child's external life. The aplomb with which some children walk out of a 'wrecked' therapy session into the rest of an uneventful day soon persuades a therapist of this truth. I cannot count the number of times I have attended Child in Care Reviews dreading the feedback about a child who has got worse and worse in our sessions only to hear how extremely well they are doing at home and school these days. Therapy often captures the distressed part of a child and frees their life for other more positive experiences.

Reconciling different points of view

Some therapies are contra-indicated because the adults have incompatible ideas. Sometimes the children themselves have other ideas when they are of an age that makes going against their will untenable. Sometimes there is no reason that therapist and child can find for embarking on what is often a long and difficult journey.

Ten-year-old Therèse was referred to me because her moroseness worried her foster mother and social worker. It transpired that her birth mother was terminally ill and that no one had explained to Therèse the exact implications of this or when and how she would visit her mother. Her sadness was appropriate and needed to be respected by those around her who knew her and who were helping to make plans for her. She needed to be included in some of this planning instead of being sent away, as she felt it, to talk to a therapist.

Fourteen-year-old Roy had been persuaded to come to therapy by his social worker who had a keen appreciation of its merits. But Roy, although in residential care and with experience of alcoholic parents, was busy 'getting on with his life'. He was doing well at school and enjoying life at the residential unit. He had had, he felt, a lifetime of counsellors and mental health professionals who were in and out of his home trying to calm his parents' excesses. He had found his chosen confidant in one of the male residential workers and they shared sporting activities. He politely let me know that he hadn't a clue what he was meant to do with therapy and was enormously relieved by my letting him off the hook. Not every young person needs therapy to heal: some, like Roy, seem to have a good instinct for how to heal themselves.

Chapter 3

Confidentiality

The work of liaison

- internal and external links
- the need for seclusion
- aggression and its containment
- therapy and the Children Act
- suicidal ideation
- sexual, emotional and physical abuse
- child protection
- when therapists have to 'tell'

Of all the issues that tax a practising child psychotherapist, those involving confidentiality have given me the most dilemmas. If we are to work effectively with accommodated young people, therapists have to take their place in the circle of people holding the safety net. This means 'networking' and being attentive to the 'slings and arrows of outrageous fortune' which are an ongoing part of these children's lives. We need to know if a foster placement is shaky, or if a parent has gone into hospital, or if our young client has to appear in court for shoplifting next Wednesday. This means that we have to have clear lines of communication with the other involved adults and that they need access to us. Some therapists use a co-worker for this liaison role, traditionally a social work colleague. Where this is possible it can work very well, for example, where therapist and social worker are colleagues on the same community mental health team or in the same foster care agency (see, for example, Chapter 9). Social workers were generally removed on cost grounds (Berelowitz and Horne 1992) from community mental health teams with little thought about the repercussions on therapeutic work.

There are, however, some advantages when both therapist and networker roles are carried out by one person. The social work team around the accommodated child may have had little experience of therapy and need to assure themselves that the therapist is competent. They may want to learn how therapists think and work. If the therapist can only be reached through an intermediary, an unhelpful veil of secrecy and mystery can shroud the therapeutic work. If other professionals are intimidated by psychotherapists we will not be told useful things we need to know about our patients and their everyday lives. Neither will we grow in our understanding of social work practices and concerns. Does this really make our therapeutic work easier or, as I suspect of some of my more removed therapist colleagues, simply hassle-free but blind? I regard it as omnipotent to believe that 'everything can be picked up in the transference'. Not if our patients fail to tell us that their foster placement is breaking down, or that they have been caught sexually abusing another child. Children often make very bad informants about shameful episodes in their current lives. Other children will assume that we know things simply because we are grown-ups. I have yet to meet a child under the age of 12 who was as concerned about confidentiality as are some psychotherapists. Children in the main assume that the 'parents' and their substitutes talk together. We should know and let the child know that we are aware of what is happening in their lives. With accommodated children I believe this is essential.

Information should flow into the therapist but what about information out? This is decidedly trickier. Psychotherapy needs a secluded time in which ideas can be talked out, played out, investigated, felt, thought over, visited from different angles, attacked, worried over, yelled at, defended against, projected out, introjected in. It is a key aspect of this process that if it is to work and the child is to allow her- or himself to venture into these dangerous emotional areas that there should be no repercussions. At least no external repercussions and certainly no tale-telling from the therapist back to mum or dad or the teacher. With no repercussions children in therapy begin to realise that this encounter is one where they can take chances. They experience the emotional containment the therapist offers during the session and they experience a lack of external consequences for their behaviour or attitude within the session. This leaves them more open to concentrate on the internal consequences.

Liam: the 3-year-old king of the castle

I once saw a very young lad who was treated rather harshly and inattentively by his also young and angry mother. She complained of his utter destructiveness and temper tantrums. She showed the health visitor the torn wallpaper, splintered skirting-boards and broken toys in his bedroom where, it was suspected, he was locked in when she had 'had enough of him'. He was found a place in a day nursery and mother was given social work help but, six months later, his destructiveness seemed unremitting.

I therefore took him on for once-weekly sessions to see if he could be helped back onto a course of development so that he would eventually cope at school. I remember his sessions vividly because they were so repetitive that they appeared seamless. He would come quietly into the room. Unable to play, he mainly poked at things or opened cupboards or shuffled items about. He carried things from one side of the room to the other in a fairly aimless way, but with increasing vehemence. Then he would drop things, bang things, throw things. This would have a rising note of provocation and aggression to it. Ultimately he would be shouting, stamping his feet, clashing things together, stockpiling a mass of items into a kind of ceremonial heap. I would have to limit some of this: 'Not the doll's house, Liam, it's too big', 'Be careful with the cup, it could break and be sharp'. On good days he would circle the pile, shouting odd phrases, 'No!', 'Get in there!', plus a wide-ranging chorus of swear words. At some point he would disagree with one of my limits and we would struggle, often physically, and at some point he would demand to be let out of the room and kick the door and anything else that threatened to stop him. I often let him go early. To not do so would have felt too punishing as I guessed he feared my retaliation. I saw him in a room in a social services day-care centre he attended so that he had only to be returned to another part of the building. Nevertheless he never refused to return and came each time cheerfully. I tried to reach him in various ways, the most successful being perhaps when I described his game as 'I'm the king of the castle, you're the dirty rascal'. Once in a while he would happily shout this back at me and sometimes he would grin a wonderfully wicked smile full of mischief. But he mainly repeated over and over his 'robber baron' game, only marginally, it seemed, accepting my existence as someone to be looted and kept out with a barricade. I spoke energetically over this crescendo of abuse, trying to describe his actions and feelings in words. I spoke of a war between a baby and a mummy where the baby was now a robber who was determined to take what he wanted. I also spoke of the baby's inability to use what he robbed without a mummy to help him. He largely ignored me. When he returned to the nursery, however, he recomposed himself. Gradually his behaviour in the nursery improved, mother was learning less punitive ways of managing him at home, his social worker relaxed when his face lost its watchful scowl and became more carefree and smiling. But in his therapy he never ceased looting, banging, stockpiling, shouting and largely ignoring me. It is true that he stayed longer, gradually, in his sessions and instead of kicking said, 'I go now.' At age 4, after a year of once-weekly sessions, he had the chance to go into a nursery class attached to the school and I believe he made a good transfer into mainstream education. He left me without a backward glance and I thought he must have been pleased to have projected his fury and anger into me and run away quickly before he supposed that I could give it back to him. I imagined I was quite a bad figure in his mind. However, years later, as I was stopped at traffic lights, a beaming face appeared at my car window. 'It's me, Mrs Hunter, Liam!' he laughed. He was seven and he recognised me before I had noticed him. He was evidently delighted to see me again. We chatted for a few moments about his school and his friends. He seemed totally sure that we were old friends.

The point of the story in this context, however, is that it was important to let Liam's accumulated anger and aggression be expressed harmlessly in his therapy. Neither the nursery nor his mother really needed to know about this. Liam could move away from this re-enactment of early battles with his mother and develop a better relationship with her. Meanwhile his anger and despair had a place where it could be expressed, understood and contained. Therapy as catharsis is not what one aims for. It is safer to continue therapy until what has been projected out has been soothed, understood and taken back in. I would not advocate 'dump and run' as a process. But as part of the therapeutic encounter it is often what we first receive and what children need to express. The gradual taking control of such behaviour and the growth of responsibility for it are better places at which to stop treatment.

Liam's sessions were angry, physical, controlling scenarios. But they were nothing that a patient child psychotherapist could not endeavour to understand and contain. I think Liam benefited from the gap between his therapy and other parts of his life and the lack of consequences from his sessions to his everyday struggles. Therapy occurs in this 'between' world which for children is usually filled with play – activities halfway between thoughts in the internal world and actions in the external world.

Steven: suspicion of sexual abuse

But what if the scenario occupying the therapeutic session looks like the following? Steven arranged the doll's house swiftly in a mood of serious attentiveness. 'Mum sits downstairs, she's knitting and watching telly. This girl is upstairs, this is her room. This boy is in the bathroom. He's going to sneak up on his sister's room.' He places a little girl doll in the bed. He puts an adult male doll in with her. He stands the brother doll in the doorway of the sister and man in bed.

MH: 'I don't understand,' I say. 'Who's that sharing the sister's bed?'
Steven: 'Don't ask!' he says, looking giggly and excited.
MH: 'Is he a boy?'
Steven: 'No . . . . a man.'
MH: 'The man is in bed with the little girl?'
Steven: 'They're just cuddling.'
MH: 'The sister looks quite small,' I say, thinking of his 13-year-old sister.
Steven: 'She's thirteen.'
MH: 'What does she think about this cuddle?'
Steven: 'She doesn't like it. She's going to wet the bed.'
MH: 'What about the boy watching?'
Steven: 'He's going to hide – he's running away.'
MH: 'I don't understand though. Where did that man come from?' (Silence)
MH: 'He's a grown up?'
Steven: 'Yep!'
MH: 'Who is he?' (Silence)
MH: 'And he's in bed with a little girl? That isn't where a grown-up man should be. What does her mum think?'
Steven: 'She's drinking wine, so she didn't hear them. The boy's flooding the bathroom – all the water is going to come down the stairs – the house is all wet – the boy's falling out of the side of the house – here's the ambulance – get in – the driver is going all skidding – oh, he's drunk – crash! That's enough of that game . . .'

He moves to another side of the room and refuses to talk more about the doll's house game. Instead he plays out a story of 'Super Snail' which he makes with Plasticine. The snail has long antennae which he shows me can get bigger or smaller. The snail leaves a wet nasty trail behind it and he laughs excitedly, showing me it falls on people and 'slimes them'.

This extract comes from my first individual session with ten-year-old Steven, living at home at this point in time with social work support to help his single mother with her four children. Given his diagnosis of learning difficulties his presentation was that of a younger child. Nevertheless my instincts in this session were that he was telling me about a real-life incident, the sexual abuse of his sister within their home. The intensity of the play, the particular answers to my questions were so different in quality from those of a child who is making up a story as it pleases him or occurs to him. These aspects gave me an inner alarm that what I was hearing was not a game. I should think few practitioners would think it right that I simply 'contain' this emotional material. And yet it is not quite a 'disclosure', and Steven was not giving me permission to take it up in the real world. In fact, he tried to move away from the story and it may well have been less explicit if I had not asked the crucial question, 'Who is that sharing the sister's bed?' It is relevant that this was the only play figure that he did not name or verbally acknowledge. I think it is likely that, despite his intentions to move away from this game which became flooded with anxiety his 'Super Snail' alternative quickly became invested with the same idea. There is a preoccupation with penis-like appendages and the idea that slimy stuff comes out of the snail and messes up people. All the play in this session is consistent with the probability that Steven has seen someone sexually abusing his sister.

Had this session occurred prior to the Children Act of 1989 there would have been more debate as to the correct actions of a child psychotherapist witnessing this material. Since then, however, the law has clearly demarcated the responsibilities of any professional toward a child at risk of significant harm. We know that sexual abuse causes children significant harm (Mullen *et al.* 1993: 721). The Act clarified that professionals must inform social services departments when such issues arise so that investigation and assessment of risk can be undertaken. To that extent it was not my task within this session to determine whether sexual abuse had occurred or not.

At the time I was with Steven I was sure that he was telling me about a real incident that had upset him and which he was communicating to me. I remember my heart sinking with the implication that I would have to do something about this. I did not relish the prospect of a child protection investigation. Yet, looking now at the evidence I had, I can see that it is far from clear what was fantasy and what, if any, reality. In his play the boy flooded the house, the boy fell out of the house, the ambulance driver was drunk. All of these parts of his play I took as metaphors for his state of mind: his feeling angry and flooded with emotion, his wish to run away from home mixed in with an idea that his home was ruined, his hope for rescue spoiled by the idea that adults get drunk and are not to be trusted. Yet I took literally the little girl cuddling in bed with the man whilst the boy watched. I did not, however, have only the evidence that can be written down here. I had Steven in the room with me, his gestures, his eyes catching mine, his body language, his emotionality. I had a communication of alarm and a request for help from him that was beyond words. Beyond or perhaps beneath words. We are, after all, animal, and our instincts for danger and communication of alarm are likely to be well honed. My conviction at that time was visceral – a gut feeling rather than intellectual. This will not do in a court of law, of course, nor is it proper evidence of abuse. Nor should it be. It relies too heavily on my being accurate in appraising this child's communications and it relies too heavily on data that I cannot replicate or put before others. It is nevertheless part of what I, as a therapist, rely on and have learned to trust. I therefore did discuss this material with Steven's mother and report it to the duty social worker.

Subsequently Sharon, Steven's 13-year-old sister, told us that she had been sexually abused by mother's boyfriend. At her request I sat with her during the disclosure interview conducted by a calm and encouraging woman PC from the Police Child Protection Team. 'I've heard about rape before,' Sharon said, 'and I thought it would be a man just jumping on a girl very suddenly. It wasn't like that. Every time I saw him he did a bit more. Sometimes I would sit on the bus in the morning and wonder could it be happening? It was so sort of gradual.'

Issues of child protection tore up the old assumptions of confidentiality. These issues brought into focus the fact that our clients are children, that our duty of care towards them is different from that towards adults in psychotherapy. A child cannot give 'informed consent' for a sexual relationship. Neither can they give 'informed consent' for keeping such a relationship secret. We cannot therefore pass to the child the burden of whether or not to keep certain confidences. Sadly our system does burden children with the traumatic and unequal task of being chief witnesses against adult abusers. I think our duty of care in this event is not to become over-zealous in the prosecution of abusers. It can nonetheless be therapeutic for children to be heard, taken seriously, and for powerful adults to make clear that they have a right to be treated respectfully. In this example Steven refused to be interviewed by the police and I advocated his right to refusal. He continued in psychotherapy with me for a year after this time and seemed to settle back into 'sessions without repercussions', that is, confidential sessions. Sharon eventually insisted on being accommodated away from home and refused to give further evidence against the abuser, who was never prosecuted. The abusive boyfriend had moved out of the home by the time of the disclosure and never returned, but mother's attitude to him remained ambivalent, and her belief in her daughter equivocal.

So much perhaps for the 'sequestered space' of a therapeutic relationship. A therapist in the midst of a child protection investigation can feel, like the child, that intimacy and privacy have been invaded and bruised by the necessities of legal and safety procedures and personnel. It is necessary but not pleasant.

These examples are at the extremes of a therapist's situation in regard to confidentiality. Alarming though the issues relating to child sexual abuse are, our actions and responsibilities are now clear-cut. I wish this were so in relation to other dilemmas.

Marianne: a risk of suicide

I think, for example, of Marianne, a 17-year-old girl in foster care. Marianne had one of those long chequered histories in and out of 'care' which makes depressing reading. Her alcoholic mother had never really been able to provide a home continuously for her and she had progressed through a dismal sequence of broken fostering arrangements and institutional care. She had skirmishes with the Juvenile Justice System for theft and property damage, including six months in a secure unit. When she was 16 she had been accommodated by a foster family within a fostering agency. This had respite care, education, therapy and various other supportive systems built in. Here, against the odds, Marianne had settled down and now planned to catch up on her education at a nearby college. She was becoming depressed, however, in proportion perhaps to the amount of time she was now spending quietly rather than drinking and 'clubbing'. She asked to see a therapist, someone she could speak to confidentially.

I visited this fostering agency once a week where I was able to see a few children in individual therapy.

Marianne impressed me as an articulate young woman who was making a determined effort to turn her life around. She presented herself well for the first ten minutes of our meeting but gradually dissolved into tears. Her depression was quite severe and I had to change my usual attitude of simply listening and 'gathering up the transference' (see Glossary) to a more active practical role of determining her mental state. For example, I asked her if she had been thinking about suicide and when she said 'yes' I investigated how far she had planned this. She told me that she thought she might take a lot of paracetamol from the bathroom cabinet one night so that she did not have to wake up in the morning.

At this juncture my main concern was to ensure her safety. She was insistent that no one should know how badly she was feeling. She did not want her foster parents to know. My impression was that this was because she felt she was a nuisance. She did not want to go to her GP or to a psychiatrist as she said that she did not want tablets. She did not want a fuss made.

I had the dilemma then of trying to decide what I should do next. Had I been able to see her the next day or every couple of days I may have opted for this course. But I only worked at this centre once a week. Had I known Marianne a little better perhaps I could have gauged how impetuous or otherwise she usually was. I gave the dilemma back to her, asking her how I could know she would be safe until next week. If she had a bad night and was again unable to sleep what would stop her taking the paracetamol from the bathroom cabinet? She could not reassure me that she would definitely not do so. I said that I needed her foster carers to keep her safe until I saw her again and I gradually persuaded her to let me tell them.

This course of action too was not without risks. I may have alienated her from me, the one source of help in whom she was willing to confide. I may have scared her more than was appropriate by warning her, as I chose to, of liver and brain damage from even a non-fatal dose of paracetamol. Instead of containing her anxieties I was in this way amplifying them. It is at these points in time that I remind myself that psychoanalytic training is an addition to ordinary common sense, it is not instead of it. Common sense tells me that a teenager who confides that she may take an overdose wants to be helped to not take it, however much she may grumble.

I did talk to Marianne's foster carers who removed the paracetamol and spent more time with her until I could see her again. Gradually we re-established a confidential boundary as I made clear that only when she was at risk would I need to let her foster carers know. Her depression eased. About six months into her therapy she suddenly rounded on me as to whether I would always be telling other people what she told me. I explained again that the only things I took outside the session were those which were connected to her current safety. I would never do this behind her back. After an angry pause she told me that something had happened to her in the past – would I be telling? I checked that neither she nor others were in danger in the present, and she confirmed this. In a changed voice she then revealed being gang-raped at the age of 14 by a group of boys she had met, one of whom she had known and liked. She had not told anyone about this rape, partly blaming herself for being in the young man's flat and for failing to act on the danger she sensed. It was a heart-breaking story. We discussed it over several months and the details were so strongly conveyed to me that I could not always hide my distress. In this way she revisited this horrible event with me and we looked at it together and mourned.

Marianne needed this story to remain confidential and under her own control. Most of us would feel the same about intimate details of our lives. She belatedly went to a doctor to have a physical check-up. Then gradually she put it aside and we went on. I sometimes feel dissatisfied with the lack of privacy for young people in care where details of their life can be on too frequent or too obvious display. Certainly the fact that we may need to know things about these children should not exonerate us from using our knowledge discreetly and with respect.

It is on the other hand difficult, as a member of the care team around a young woman like Marianne, to not share the understanding that some of her behaviour is linked to past experiences.

Marianne was often hostile toward men. She had difficulty with boyfriends and difficulties confiding in her foster carers. She believed that others may see in her something disgusting, something shameful, something that caused her to be denigrated and raped. It is the bitter product of this kind of experience that what is put into the victim is not just the penis but shame. This shame rightfully belongs to the perpetrator. In rape, the massive power of 'projective identification' is laid bare. The perpetrator bullies and depersonalises his victim, evacuating into her his own hatred and disgust in erotic and triumphant form. The perpetrator walks away in a state of denial and self-justification. In the victim are to be found the feelings which logically belong to the perpetrator: disgust, despair, shame, self-doubt. Added to the physical trauma and fear of annihilation there enters into the victim a psychological trauma, a vision of herself as contemptible. It is this which the therapist and victim can address and reformulate. Partly the process is one which parallels the mother–infant relationship of early days. The baby in its bodily messes is soothed and cleaned. Psychologically the mother gives the baby a perception of self that shines through any dirty nappy. The child is affirmed as lovable. So the process in therapy examines and soothes the various fears of being disgusting. The therapist affirms the victim as lovable.

These intimate conversations deserve a high degree of privacy and tact. They are appropriately confidential.

William: physical punishment

Occasionally it has happened that a child I am seeing turns up with a non-accidental injury or tells me that 'mum hit me with the electric cable' or 'dad got out the belt'. These all present dilemmas about a psychotherapist's appropriate course of action. I think I used to be less aware of discussing such incidents with a duty social worker and probably let many of them just go by. My experience of therapy with William, though, alerted me to the possibility that a child can be being severely and routinely beaten whilst only giving partial information and hints to concerned adults.

William was already under a Full Care Order when he began therapy with me when he was 10. He had recently been fostered following a severe beating from his well-built mother. Once in the safety of a foster family he let it be known that he did not want to go home. The involvement of social services had been lengthy, since William's birth, in fact, to his 18-year-old mother whose parents refused to support her with the baby. However, the fact that she had stuck by her baby despite periods of foster care seemed to speak for an enduring relationship. There was little on his record of abusive incidents yet the relationship between mother and son was correctly perceived as not very good and, following the birth of a sister, William was clearly scapegoated by mother. Father had left before his birth and mother lived alone with the two children.

Over the six years of his therapy I came to understand retrospectively what life at home had been like for William. After the birth of his sister, his mother had blamed and punished William for anything that went wrong in the household. When he began to tell me about the beatings it was always in relation to some housework he had not done properly or something that had got broken or his clumsiness or 'stupidity'. He therefore felt he was somewhat to blame, although even at 10 years of age he felt his mother 'went over the top'. He often stayed away from school until the injuries healed. He made up excuses as to why he could not undress and invented reasons for his cut lips and bruised face. Most of the time he feared his mother's anger to such an extent that he dared not tell: she would surely hurt him even more. Once when he was in the bath she held him under the water, saying she would drown him. He lived in absolute fear of her. He did, however, from time to time, let various people know that he was being hurt. A teacher at school was told. A boyfriend of his mother's saw him beaten. His half-sister's dad sympathised with him and told his mother to be less severe. William told a social worker that he was sometimes hit. William never protested too loudly or too assertively. He thought he was probably a bad boy and he was not sure what he deserved. He was ashamed of being so bad that he got beaten. It was his little sister who eventually told her teacher that mum had pounded William's head against the wall and kicked him down the stairs.

William was surprised that he had the right to not be assaulted. He was grateful to be in a foster home and not to have to return home. Much later he had the recurrent fantasy of going home and beating up his mother. Even at 15 years of age he would wake trembling and sweating in the night in the middle of a flashback that he was at home and about to be beaten.

Some adults in William's life knew that he was hit. He had told a social worker years before. His class teacher knew. But everyone assumed that it was not severe. No one interfered.

When another child, 7-year-old Lewis, after missing one session arrived at the next with a recovering but badly split lip because 'dad smacked him', I let his mother know that I would be telling social services. Months later his father, who had been warned about his physical violence, put the boy into the boot of his car and drove him around 'to teach him a lesson'. Some parents are so astray in their ideas of acceptable ways to treat children that we may lack the imagination to comprehend it or to guess that it is happening. Psychotherapists are not in a position to get the full picture of a child's situation and we are in the difficult position of perhaps ruining the trust of our patients and their parents. Whilst there are children in the situation of William and Lewis, however, there is no better option than letting our social work colleagues know. It is a betrayal of trust to not tell.

Charlotte: return to mother

I met 7-year-old Charlotte when she was living in a local authority community home. Because of the severity of her difficulties she was considered unsuitable to be fostered and her future seemed set for a lifetime of institutional care. Her single mother had three other children to cope with, all boys, but felt that Charlotte was too much for her to handle. On several occasions Charlotte was 'received into care' but was always removed without warning by her mother. The local authority and mother became embattled and finally the local authority insisted on a Full Care Order and residential accommodation which they were awarded after a lengthy court case. Charlotte was a physical, hysterical girl who teased and bit and hit out without control or remorse. I saw her three times a week for four years (see Chapter 6 for an account of this therapy).

Towards the end of our third year, Charlotte's mother made a strong bid to have her daughter returned home to her. I was in the uncomfortable position of knowing a great deal about the abusive experiences this child had suffered. She had been sexually abused by mother's boyfriend. She had witnessed mother and boyfriend having sexual intercourse. She had been hit, and locked in her bedroom for so long that she had urinated on the floor. She had seen this boyfriend break into their home and assault mother. At the age of 7 she could describe vaginal intercourse and anal intercourse. She knew about semen and how it differed from urine. She could mimic female orgasm. She could mimic male penetration.

In Charlotte's games the crying baby was always dropped and forgotten in exciting chases which involved kidnap and sex. She portrayed a mother who fought tooth and nail to have her children, only carelessly to deliver them into the hands of a monster or to lock them into a cupboard cold and hungry. In Charlotte's games there was a remorseless, endless cycle of escape, capture, abuse, rescue, recapture, abuse, abuse, abuse. From inside the 'cold cupboard' or from 'under the sex blanket', Charlotte would 'telephone' me asking me to come and get her away from a monster who was 'sexing' her. I would ask her what should I reply on the phone. She told me, 'Say you can't come this year but you will come next year.'

To add to my difficulties with confidentiality the original social work team that brought Charlotte into accommodation was reorganised so that new social workers then took over the case. As happens very often with transferred cases a lot of information known informally but not documented was lost. A lot of documented information was ignored and disowned. I became the person with the fullest memory of Charlotte's past: indeed neither Charlotte nor I could escape from it.

In this situation it cannot be right for a child psychotherapist to refuse to participate in plans for the child's future. The best interests of the child dictate that the judge who will make a decision about future placement should have access to relevant information known about the child by her therapist. Of course, it makes future therapy extremely difficult. Charlotte by now was enjoying access visits with her mother although she became depressed before them and wild and unmanageable after them. Her mother refused to acknowledge her daughter's abuse and refused to work with the local authority. She simply wanted Charlotte back. Over a lengthy trial I put before the court my evidence for believing that Charlotte would not be protected in her mother's care. This meant that I opposed Charlotte's mother and made Charlotte's relationship to me one of divided loyalties. Of course, I did not characterise my testimony to Charlotte as being 'against mum'. But her mother did. Charlotte came into a session following an access visit and sobbed her heart out because her mother told her I was preventing her going home. 'My mum don't like you,' she sobbed, 'and you hate my mum.'

Therapy with abused children has to take place in a very clear framework of child protection and the best interests of the child. This on occasion clashes with the best interests of a therapeutic relationship which has to give way for the child's overall good.

During the assessment process I state clearly to children the aims and the limits of my confidentiality. I explain that therapy is essentially a private relationship where I must think about what they tell me and not tell others without their permission. Of course, they may talk about therapy to others. But – and I always emphasise this 'but' – I would 'tell' if they were likely to come to harm or if others were likely to be harmed without my telling.

A boy of 14 who was accused of but denied sexually interfering with his 3-year-old sister kept on asking me about the exact limits of my confidentiality. My unvoiced assumption was that he wanted to tell me of his guilt but feared that I would tell his social worker and others. Although I was able to talk through the various possibilities and what they may feel like, although I stressed the need for a person to face up to their actions and get help to control themselves, I could not assure him of my silence. He quickly denied his interest in the dilemma and gradually withdrew from therapy. I did wonder whether he may have confided and gained the help and courage to tell others if he could have been assured of confidentiality. But duty of care extended to smaller children in his home and it was necessary to agree with the social work decision to foster him in a home without vulnerable younger children.

Confidentiality should not be a cloak for collusion nor an excuse for therapists not to shoulder ordinary adult responsibilities in relation to children. Nevertheless it is always difficult and debatable where exactly to draw the line. A therapeutic relationship necessarily involves trust of the therapist. Sometimes children have to be told that this trust extends to the therapist's judgement to share things with others.

Chapter 4

Joseph – a therapy in pictures

The effects of neglect and abuse

- confidentiality and duty of care
- defences of denial and omnipotence
- resilience
- siblings in therapy
- interpreting children's pictures
- super-heroes
- transference
- projection of unwanted feelings
- denial and mistrust
- progress in therapy
- partnership
- therapeutic gains

Joseph was 6 years old when we first met. An earnest, fast-moving boy with little, round, wire-rimmed glasses that gave him an endearing look. He talked quickly and indistinctly and his eyes darted everywhere. Hungry for attention and affection he was immediately and too quickly close enough to hug me, which he did awkwardly. He talked easily and confusedly about his best friend, Thomas, about his sister, Donna, about his mum, about other children in the 'children's home', about his pleasure that I wanted to see him. The staff of the home had told him that I was good at helping children with worries and that I had loads of toys, he said. He looked about him happily and soon decided that he would draw a picture. When I asked him after a short while whether he had worries that I could help with he said, 'No, nothing worries me at all!' After a pause, he added, except his sister Donna being sad. He did not like that. She cried sometimes. She did not like Darren shouting at her. I had to ask him who Darren was and he answered simply, 'Who lives with mummy.' Later he added, 'Don't tell.' His drawing was immediately a narrative one.

I explained to him in simple words the limits of my confidentiality, my duty of care toward him and other children. He reluctantly accepted that I would help to protect him and his sister by telling people who would help.

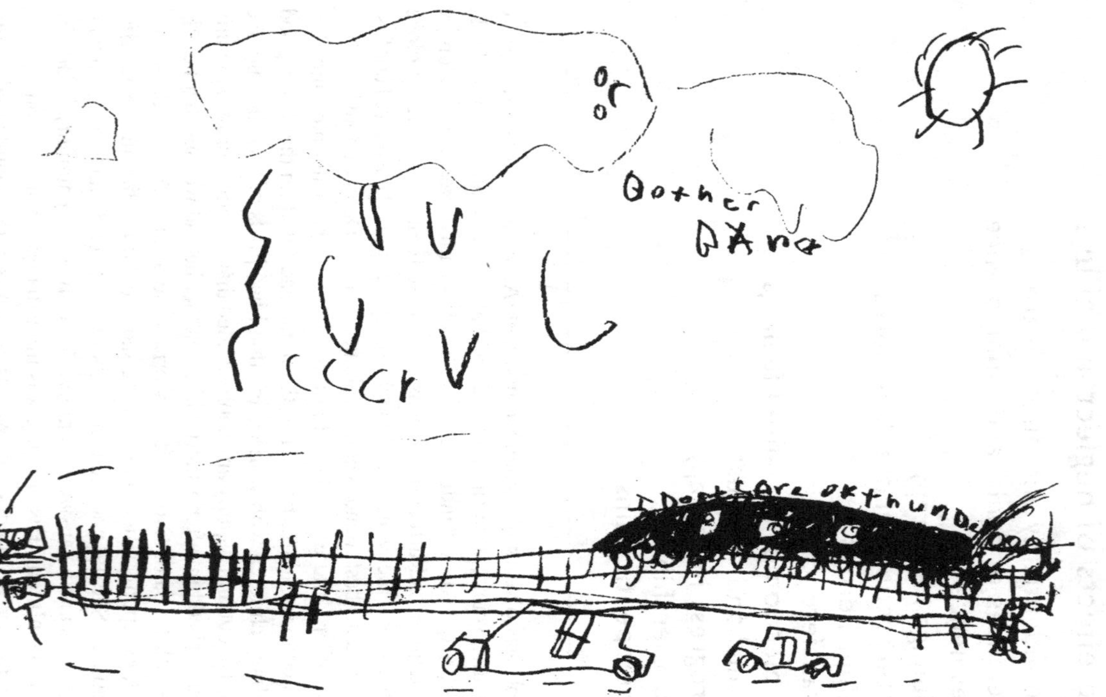

Figure 1 A train heading toward a road crossing

His first picture (Figure 1) showed a train heading toward a road crossing. He called the train 'Thomas'. A boy was on the train. There was a storm. The clouds were banging together. It was thunder. He wrote the words 'Bother. Bang' near the clouds. He drew what he called 'grumpy face' on one big cloud. It was raining and sending lightning bolts down, just where the train would soon be passing.

I wondered aloud whether the train passengers would get wet. Or hear the thunder. Or see the lightning. It looked a bit frightening, I said.

He chuckled and told me, 'He doesn't care! He isn't afraid.' He wrote on top of the train, 'I don't care. OK. Thunder!'

Despite his words his anxiety seemed high at this point and he jumped down from his seat at the table and found the box of toy cars. He continued to push toy cars up and down the room until it was time to leave.

Whilst he was on the floor and I remained at the table looking at his picture I asked about Thomas. Was that his friend? Was he the boy on the train? Joseph had told me his best friend was Thomas.

'No, he's not on the train, he's Thomas – the Tank Engine!' Joseph exclaimed. 'That's my best friend.'

How often it is that the child before me seems lively, friendly, full of energy, optimism and affection. And yet the history tells the most appalling tale. Some of this is the child's capacity to deny and to split off feelings. Some of it is the child's resilience and capacity to maximise good experiences despite other bad experiences (Fonagy *et al.* 1992: 231).

Joseph had been brought into a residential home three months before our meeting. He and his sister were the subjects of care proceedings for severe neglect. His 8-year-old sister, Donna, had disclosed sexual abuse by more than one perpetrator, at different times in her life.

The children's history was one of shuttling between their separated father's and mother's care. It transpired that they had been sexually abused by a boyfriend of their mother, by a friend of their father and by a neighbour. These abuses compounded their lack of protective parenting and made patent their vulnerability. Their removal from both parents after eight years had been appallingly overdue. One of the difficulties that face social services departments is tracking such children. Their parents continually moved, their domestic arrangements were fluid and Joseph and Donna had learnt not to complain.

Children with Donna and Joseph's experiences learn to be extremely careful about trusting adults with information that might incriminate them or rebound on them. Outwardly placatory and happy, they hide their thoughts with the skill of diplomats in dangerous, foreign territory.

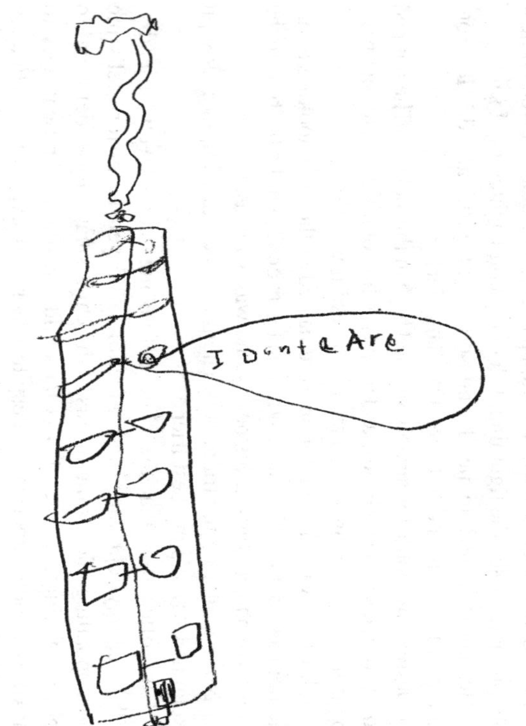

Figure 2 Empire State Building

I saw Joseph twice-weekly for three years and nine months before he and his sister were adopted together. His sister Donna I referred for therapy elsewhere but, when after a year she was still not receiving therapeutic help, I also took her into therapy twice-weekly with me. As a rule it is best to let siblings have their own different therapists so that they have maximum privacy, free from rivalry with siblings. It is also difficult for a therapist to listen to two different versions of the same event without being influenced by the other child's viewpoint. In a similar situation today I might suggest seeing siblings together so that these influences are apparent to both children. In the event, however, I was faced with a child who had already had a year of individual therapy whilst his sister had had none. With considerable generosity Joseph welcomed my seeing his sister. Her first sessions in therapy were characterised by detailed drawings of people waiting at bus stops. With chagrin I interpreted this to mean that she had waited and waited for her turn. Meanwhile Joseph's therapy quickened with memories and this culminated in his eventual disclosures of sexual abuse. He seemed aware that his sister might tell me before he did. It is instructive to note that it took him well over a year to begin to articulate his past abuse.

The course of many themes in Joseph's therapy can be traced through a selection of his lively, highly expressive narrative drawings. I have selected twelve of them for this purpose drawn from the whole course of his therapy and presented in the order in which he drew them, although they were many months apart.

The picture drawn on the first session (Figure 1) captures succinctly for me Joseph's preoccupation with travelling into danger. His claim that Thomas the Tank Engine was his best friend was later revealed as an actual confusion between fantasy and reality. His case notes stated that when he was 4 he had believed he was Superman. He had jumped out of his bedroom window and spent a week in hospital. Joseph's attitude to his situation of danger is also shown in his drawing. He denies that he minds or that he is fearful.

The second picture (Figure 2) comes again from the early months of therapy. At the top of the Empire State Building a fire has broken out. Below it a boy at the window claims, 'I don't care.' The peril of a boy in this situation is clear, as is his attempt to deny being afraid.

The third picture (Figure 3) is the story of an oil tanker that has hit rocks. Oil pours into the sea. Inside, a boy looks out but he has good reason to be cheerful. Superman is coming to his aid: 'Yeh, yeh, yeh,' he shouts. Although Joseph is still having to invoke a super-figure to overcome danger, there is a separation of the boy and the super-figure.

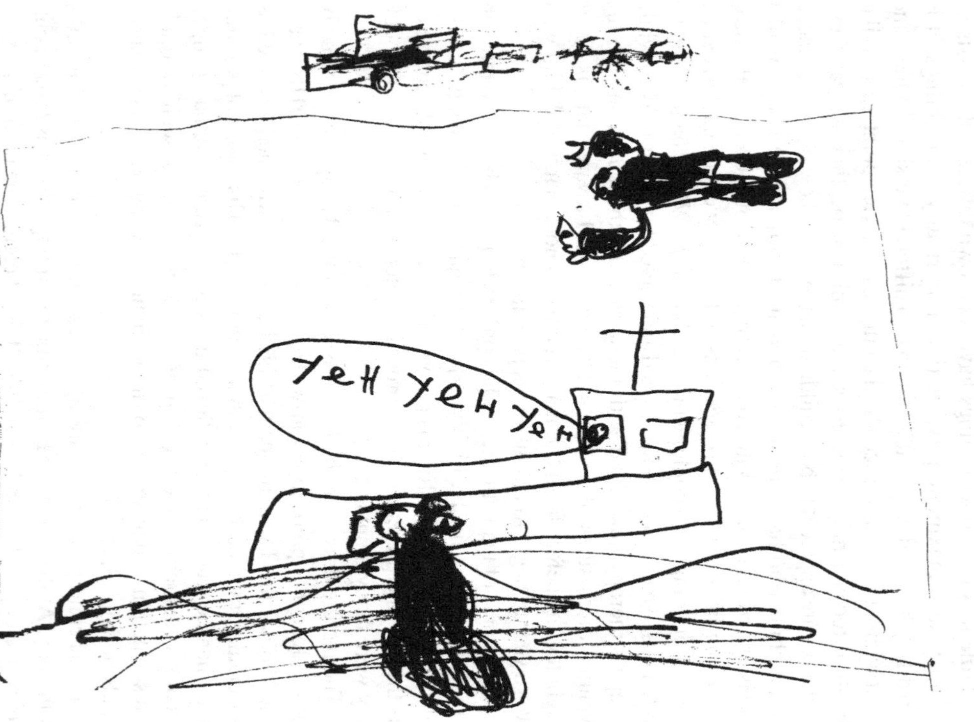

Figure 3 Oil tanker

He is still having to rely on magical omnipotent thinking to rescue him from danger but he acknowledges that he is not superhuman.

Joseph and I discussed his feelings that things were so dangerous that super-powers seemed needed to help him.

He drew the fourth picture (Figure 4) some months later. Joseph's father had a red car which Joseph admired and tried to idealise along with his father. Miserable in his mother's care, Joseph told me how his dad had come to get him. There was one frightening memorable occasion when he only took Joseph and not Donna. Donna was like a mother to Joseph. He was bereft without her. Rowing with the children's mother, their father had dragged the terrified Joseph away in his red car to his girlfriend's house a hundred miles away. Joseph was sick on the journey. His father's red car was hard for Joseph to draw, and was usually incomplete. Angry jagged shapes are involved. Huge phallic exhausts emit black fumes from both ends. Other cars beep, the driver shouts, 'Shut up, shut up.'

In looking together at this picture, Joseph and I talked about his dad. I helped him acknowledge that he admired his father's strength and virility. Harder to admit was Joseph's fear of his father's bad temper and aggressive outbursts. Joe told me that, when he himself was angry, he thought of his father and copied his words.

The fifth picture (Figure 5) comes from the second year of therapy shortly before my summer holiday. It is ingeniously detailed and the story is more complex. Joseph's dad's red car has become Joseph's own red Porsche. There is a £100 note he has just seen in the road. Ahead, a notice of road works warns of a hole. I am symbolised by the 'Alitalia' coach which Joseph says I am taking to my holiday. I am driving. This also symbolises my carrying lots of passengers. Behind the coach a Mercedes with an erect phallic shape, I think represents my rich husband. The bus is blowing smoke at it. Joseph thinks this may obscure the £100 note in the road. Above this couple a 'slimer' hovers, ready to descend. This 'slimer' is an idea from the film *Ghostbusters*. It is a ghostly slimy-green mess. I think it symbolises Joseph's fear that my husband and I will have slimy, nasty sex. In this way Joseph brings the issues from his past, now lodged in his own psyche and expectations, in his internal world, into a transference relationship with me in therapy. My pending absence is seen as an abandonment of him to danger whilst I go off with a sexual man and my children. His rivalry with my husband – both in red cars – is Oedipal. He must stop in the picture and there is a hole, a gap, ahead. He compensates himself with £100. He wants me to send away my suitor and make him miss his £100.

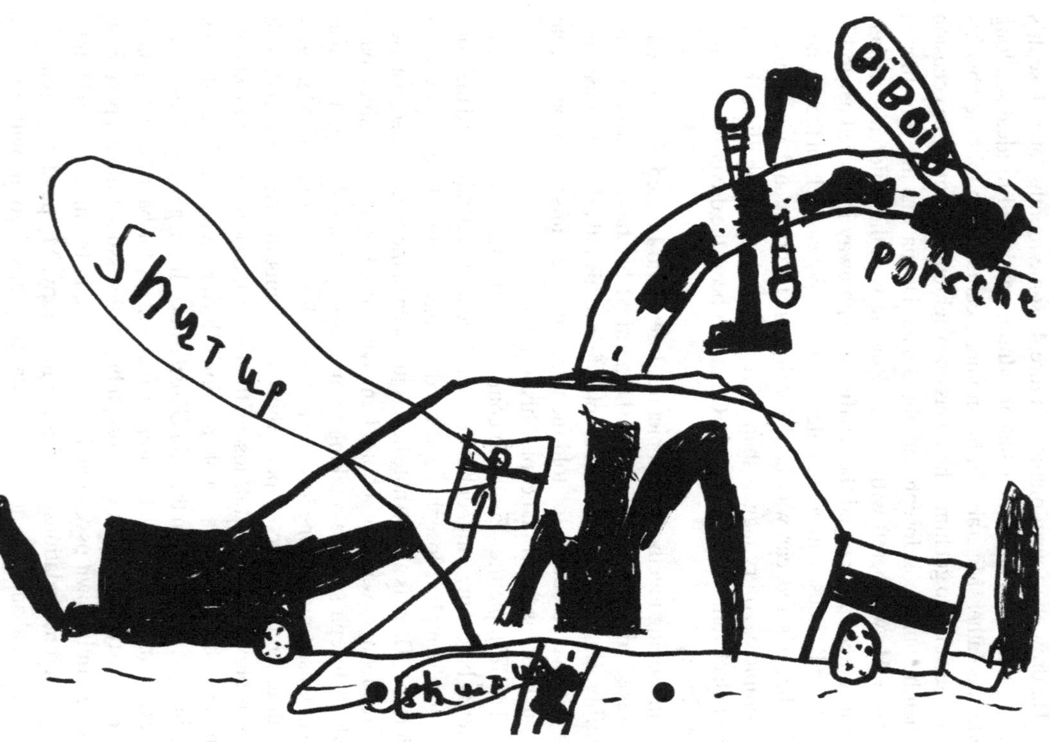

Figure 4 Car

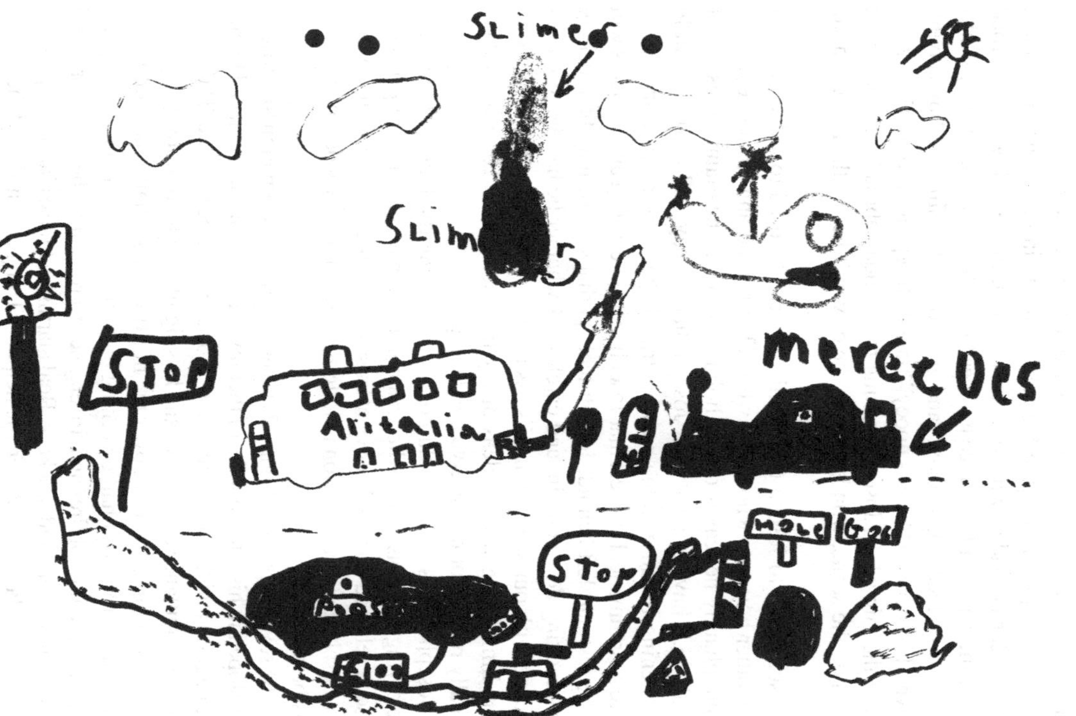

Figure 5 Porsche and Mercedes

Interpreting the picture piece by piece to Joseph means that we built up between us a shared understanding of his feelings. He would often acknowledge that I was right or he would correct me, 'No, it's not your children in the coach, it's all the others you see in here!'

The sixth picture (Figure 6) shows Joseph himself going on holiday. His red car is loaded with suitcases. Again, money blows in the road beside the car. Will Joseph see it? 'Yes I will,' he cries triumphantly whilst the car driver says 'Come on!' and gets covered in slime. A boy is lying down. 'He is crying "booy – hooey"' laughs Joseph as he draws him. He's left in the rain whilst Joseph is going to a holiday abroad. The sun looks down on the scene, wondering will he or won't he see the money in the road.

I suggested to Joseph that in this material he tried to lodge his fears in another boy, one who cried, who is left behind and whom he mocks. Triumphantly he leaves on the holiday of which he claims he is not at all afraid. I have to gently tell Joseph that he may find journeys a little frightening because in the past his travels between mother and father were so traumatic. I suggest that Joseph feels like crying and wonders will he be lost and left behind. Joseph feels perhaps that I may be mocking him, looking down on him and careless of whether he has the resources to cope with our separation. His assumption about me when I am away from him is tinged with ideas of my tantalising him. He feels he may equally receive or not receive good things.

Joseph at this point would not accept my interpretation. He thought the crying boy was a boy who was not accompanying the group abroad. Joseph relished this boy's envy at missing out. Joe was not going to look too closely at his satisfaction in lodging a part of his own deprived self in this boy.

The seventh picture (Figure 7) shows a new preoccupation that Joseph developed in his later months of therapy. The red cars are replaced by red fire engines and the hope that rescue and relief may be possible. The police car and ambulance are smaller and less significant to him. Joseph feels he needs something to cool down the hot fires of sexuality, something to rescue him from the phallic burning building of his early picture (Figure 2). These pictures of fires and fire engines were many. They also portrayed an idea of trickery and mockery. Real alarms and false alarms are present. Is someone playing a joke on the helpers? Things are not what they seem and there is no way to tell real from false. Joseph's worries about the mendacity of adults and his own disingenuous innocence came to the fore. Joseph struggled with his ambivalence about his own sexuality, which he felt was powerful, magical, omnipotent, as well as dangerous. At this point

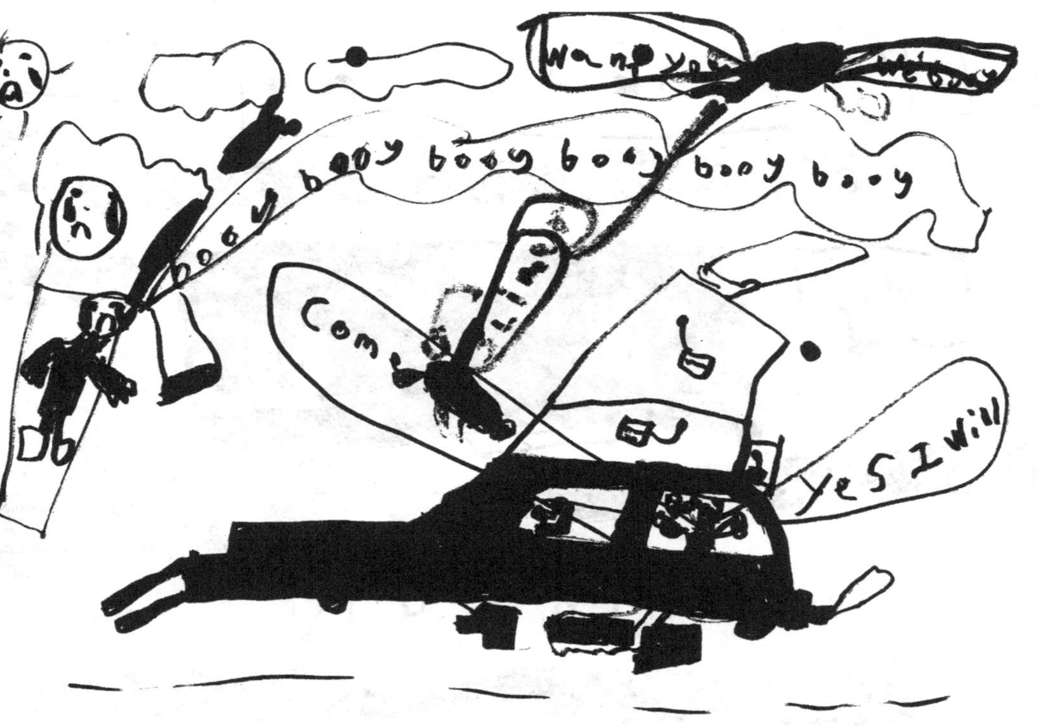

Figure 6 Car with suitcases

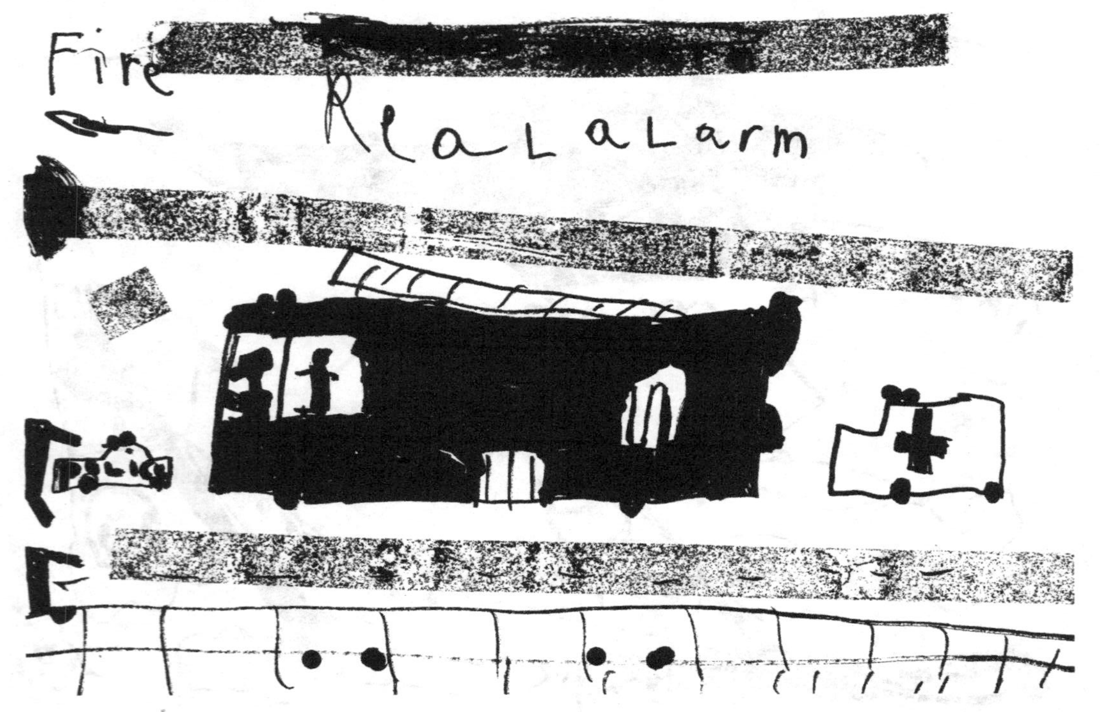

Figure 7 Red fire engine

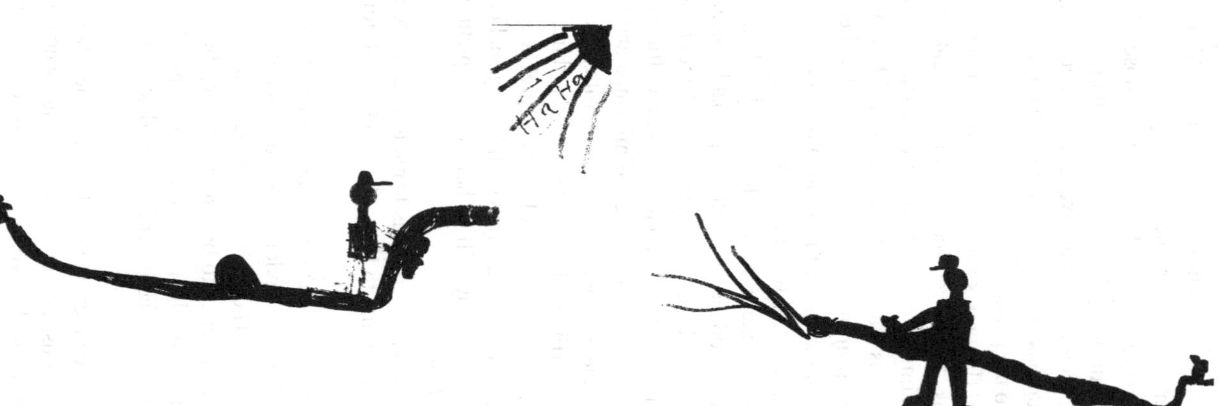

Figure 8 Man with blocked hose and sun smiling

in time he was known to be involved with other children in sexual games at the home. Joseph's strong denial of his own feelings and aggression makes it the more difficult for him to believe in truthful others. When I point this out to him he considers me with suspicion.

The fireman in Figure 8 has a blockage in his hose. Does something stop the help getting through? The sun mocks and laughs from its lofty height. The picture is comical, a real joke. The blocked hosepipe may also have sexual connotations containing the idea that something tricky and bad has happened to the penis.

Pictures 9 and 10 (Figures 9 and 10) were drawn in the same session, after a holiday break. Joseph returned from these breaks distant and full of denial, wanting simply to pour himself into activity with scarcely a glance at me. The taxi is loaded with suitcases, and I say that Joseph has the holiday very much in mind. He pushes the unfinished picture aside to redraw the shape of the car. It turns into a hearse, with a coffin where the suitcases had been. In this way I can talk to Joseph about his fear that separation between us is cause for fear that it will be final. Either he will die because he feels abandoned, or I will die, probably because of his rage at me. Joseph only gradually came to accept that I could continue to care about him despite his rivalry, his sexuality, his deceitfulness, and his rage at my absences. Nevertheless his denials diminished and I could see his anxiety diminish whenever I put these difficult truths into words.

The eleventh picture (Figure 11) is taken from the third year of therapy. A boy is drowning in the sea. Instead of 'I don't care' he is calling simply 'Help!' Above him, only inches away, a round orange helicopter is letting down a safety ladder. The boy will be helped. The picture is complete, confident, boldly coloured.

Joseph learned to acknowledge his fears, to take some responsibility for his own state, to trust and to be bold enough to ask for help. He felt that help would reach him.

More and more Joseph's pictures began to show cooperative themes. The fire in Figure 12 is now under control and being dealt with by two engines and two firemen. The feeling is balanced and contained. By this stage in therapy Joseph began to be a more trusting boy in a world that ceased to be dominated by themes of indifferent fate. Joseph and I had become a team dealing with feelings of danger, destruction and sexualised aggression.

By the time that Joseph left the residential home where I saw him, he had become a more robust boy of nearly 10 years who could engage in honest conversations about his worries. He was concerned that he might be badly treated at his new adoptive home and school. We discussed his

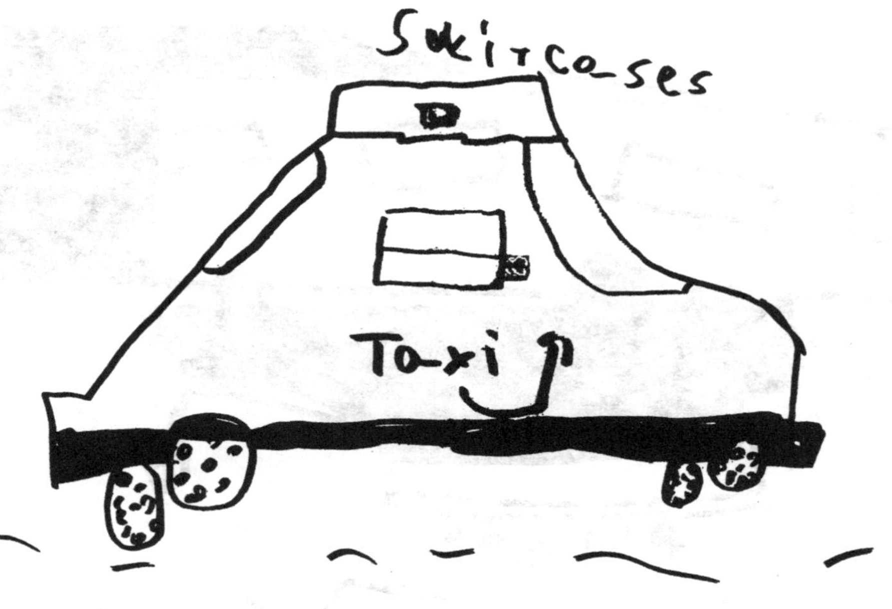

Figure 9 Taxi with suitcases

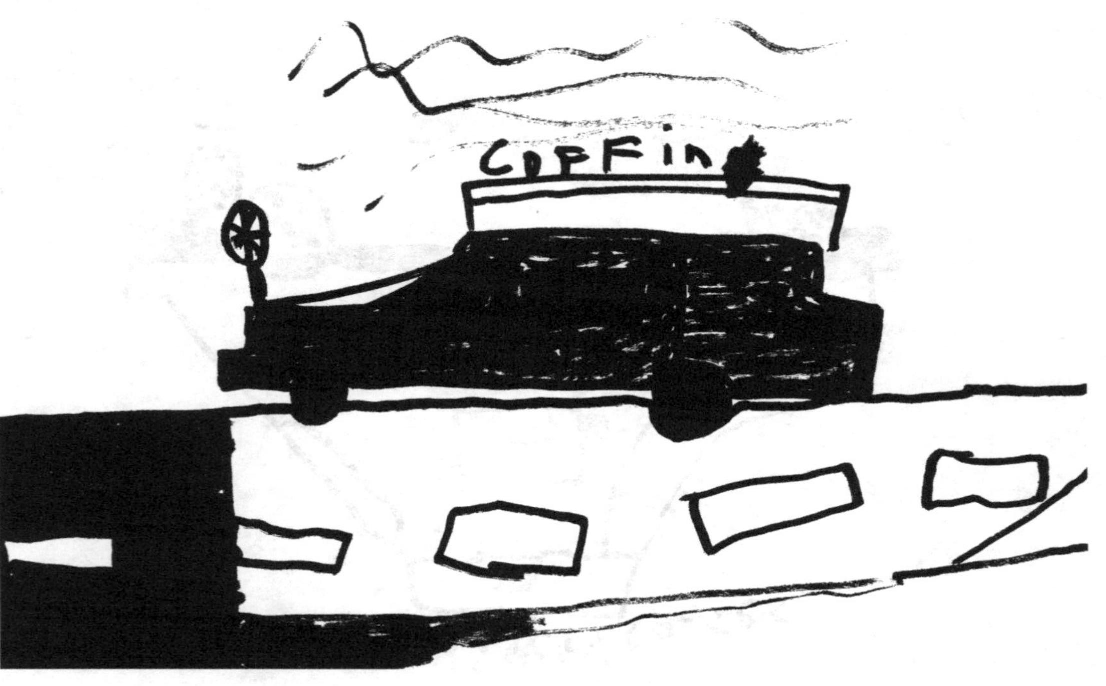

Figure 10 Coffin and hearse

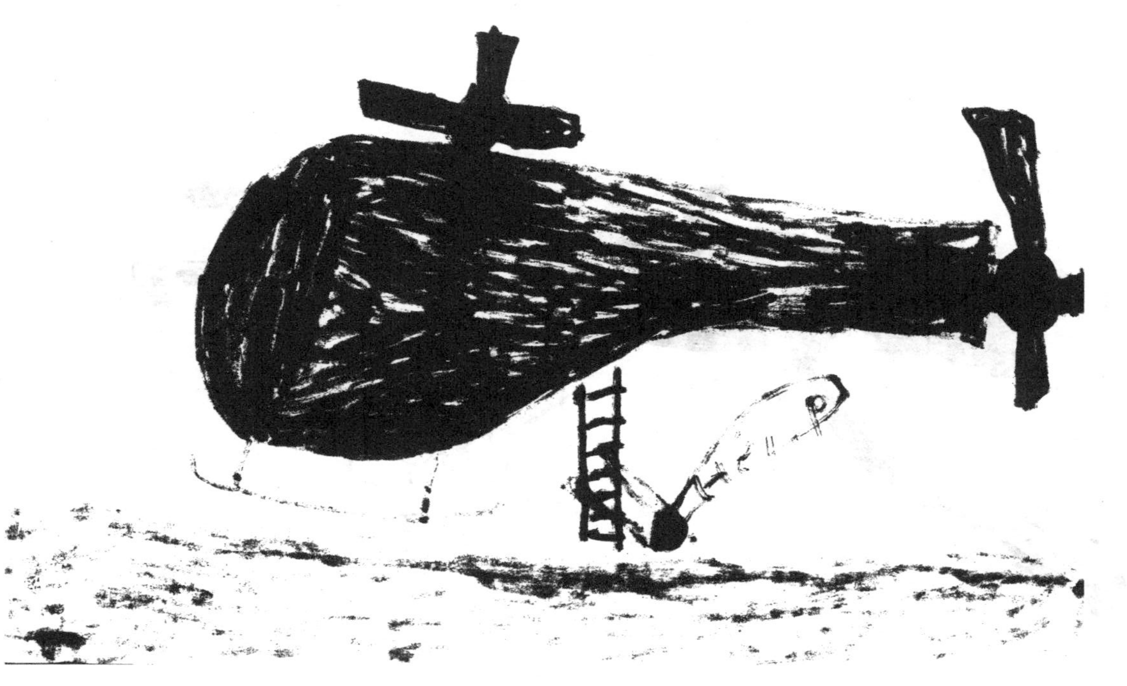

Figure 11 Helicopter and sea

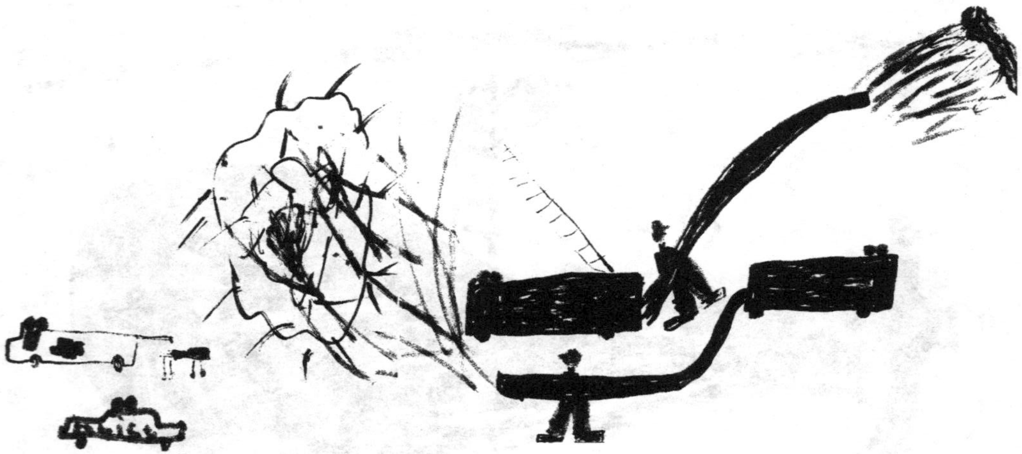

Figure 12 Two engines and two firemen

fears about himself in this future context. Joseph worried that his anger, his rivalry and his hidden aggression meant that he had deserved his abusive treatment. His estimation of himself was therefore lower than first appeared. When he and his sister left for their new home he knew at least where his fears came from and was able to question whether his new relationships had to replay past abusive relationships. He went forward with more ability to trust and ask for help.

Of course, this account of therapy is necessarily schematic and can give only a flavour of the many different conversations I had with Joseph. Therapy does not follow a steady course and there are setbacks and diversions as well as progress along the way. There were inevitably times when I was not well in touch with Joseph, when I misunderstood or misinterpreted. Through it all, the most important aspect is that one tries honestly and without preconditions to communicate, to understand and to accept the other. Joseph and I came to be good partners in therapy and we parted with sadness. His own comment on his therapy written on his goodbye card to me was 'thank you for getting all my bad feelings out'. My own view was the hope that he was better equipped to deal with his feelings.

Chapter 5

Charlotte

Early deprivation and abuse

– aggression and fear of retaliation
– body and ego boundaries
– use of the manic defence
– child's view of sexuality
– the Oedipus complex
– interpretation and containment
– rivalry and perversity
– diagnostic difficulties

After a dozen or so encounters with Charlotte I tried to take stock of the overwhelming chaos and confusion she brought into my room. I seemed to be with a small fierce animal rather than a little girl, and one that enjoyed attack, rather like a puppy will happily tussle and chew on an item you may be trying to retrieve. She was a pretty 7-year-old girl with fair wavy hair and appealing blue eyes. She looked alert and lively, for the most part using an impetuous provocative grin and often laughing or shouting loudly. By contrast she sucked her thumb frequently and could have the glazed 'tuned out' look of a 2-year-old about to fall asleep. Her vocabulary was wide and imitative. She appeared to be articulate and bright. The assumption of her cleverness derived from her provocative behaviour toward adults and her quick-wittedness in seizing opportunities for disruption. The staff in the children's home where she lived felt that she was a strong opponent, loudly and effectively promoting her own cause. She rarely expressed sadness, hurt or fear except in noisy displays which had a false attention-seeking quality to them. This is an extract from our second meeting:

> Charlotte circles the room giggling, opens cupboard doors, climbs in and out of the empty space, throwing out the blankets in the large cupboard. She suddenly rushes to the table, gets up on top of it despite my protests and grabs the curtains, jumping to the floor clutching them and ripping them in the process. I catch her awkwardly but talking calmly, trying to quieten her. She shrieks loudly and excitedly

> that she's going to wet herself and I persuade her to come to the adjoining toilet. She grabs everything in sight, throws the toilet roll into the bowl and when I am trying to remove the toilet cleaner she gets past me back into the room and proceeds to use the felt tip pens to draw on everything she can – walls, table, curtains. She is laughing and shrieking with seeming delight. Several times I offer to take her back to her carers: she does not have to stay with me if she is afraid of me. She spits and dribbles and throws things at me but refuses to leave the room . . .

This is an unusual and extreme level of chaos and provocative behaviour from a 7-year-old who had just met me.

Early sessions with Charlotte were short, as I tried to establish limits as to what I would allow in the room. Gradually this wild behaviour began to be less of an attack and more of a communication:

> . . . after several skirmishes Charlotte claims she 'will be good now' if I let her stay. She picks up a little plastic figure and then impulsively puts it into her mouth and cracks its head off with her teeth. After a fleeting look of triumph and spite she collapses with a loud roar of pain. The sharp plastic has scratched her gums. Holding her firmly I remove the pieces of plastic and talk to her about a little Charlotte who makes herself feel very big and powerful and fierce but then gets hurt and suddenly realises how small she is. She becomes calmer and asks me will I tuck her into bed 'like a baby'. She lies on the back support of the sofa, not on the seat. 'The baby's bed is on that high ledge?' I ask, disapprovingly. She is insistent, 'Yes, the baby is sleeping on a cliff.' She tells me that 'it may fall over or it may balance'. She asks me to cover her up with the blankets and I do. Uncomfortable as it must be, she puts the covers completely over her head. The baby is not to hear the thunderstorm outside, she tells me . . .

In further sessions 'the baby on the cliff' hears a mother and boyfriend arguing and trying to control a child who won't sleep, a boy who is meant to help, a dog who runs about yapping excitedly. Charlotte takes the role of each character without pause and switching from one position to another graphically to portray her scene:

> She gets out of 'bed' and runs around in a sudden brief 'skirmish' and gets back. Speaking in a changed voice that I gather is her

> mothers, she says, 'Get into that bleeding bed, Tommy. Go to sleep! Cut that out! The baby's asleep. What you got there, Felix? Done a bleedin' packet, 'ave you? Cor!' She pretends to change a nappy. 'What are you doing that for?' she replies now in a gruff man's voice. 'I'm just putting up the Christmas decorations!' She turns into a dog who yaps and bounces around. Mother's voice screams louder: 'Who let that bleedin' dog out? Hit him, Charlotte, for doing that on the carpet. Give him a right one. Get in there, Champion. Get in that b—— f—— room. Now you'll get no food for that! Justin! Put that pizza on for us! You stupid bastard, you know the oven's hot . . . If you've burnt yourself it's your own fault.'

In these early sessions the management of this wildly hyperactive girl took most of my thinking space. Thinking had to be done as I later wrote up the session and tried to digest what had been poured torrentially into me. Presumably Charlotte had no time or resources to think either when she was attacking the room or rôle-playing in this exhausting way. The little islands of calm that began to appear during her time as a baby sleeping on a cliff also seemed non-reflective time for her. The baby was as stiff and still as a corpse. Outside of this enactment, thunderstorms of a human kind seemed to rage. The contrast between the precariously balanced stiff baby and the energy and licence of the dog gave me pause for thought. Charlotte often identified with the dog in her play.

A brief history of Charlotte's life

Charlotte was the second child of her 20-year-old mother. Her father, said to be a man of limited intelligence, was with her mother for the first year of Charlotte's life. He was then committed to prison for a long prison sentence for violent crime. Mother had left the new-born Charlotte in hospital and discharged herself, the first of a series of desperate abandonings of her daughter. Depressed for much of the child's early life, her mother described Charlotte as a very quiet baby who fed and slept continually. Father and mother's relationship was unhappy and violent. Mother thought he was 'mental' and that Charlotte was just like him in the violence of her temper. Despite recorded concern for Charlotte by the staff of her nursery school, mother's volatility and Charlotte's frequent absences meant that little effective intervention occurred until she was 4. Charlotte was 'received into care' three times in her fourth year and removed each time by her mother without negotiation. At the age of 6 the allocated social worker removed Charlotte under a Place of Safety Order for physical abuse. When it was revealed that Charlotte had been sexually abused by mother's boyfriend a Full Care Order was made and an eventual Care Plan for long-term accommodation was the result. Charlotte confirmed the allegation of sexual abuse but could give no coherent account of it: for example, she also claimed that this man had cut her head completely off. Perhaps there was symbolic truth in this wild statement but there was judged to be insufficient evidence for a prosecution of this man.

What was wrong with Charlotte?

An educational assessment of Charlotte found:

> Her short-term recall memory is above average and her verbal reasoning appears to be at least within the average ability range. Her poor level of literacy and numeracy is likely to be accounted for by lack of experience and stimulation, frustrated by her behavioural problems. Her distractibility and preoccupation with her own internal world are clearly affecting her ability to learn. . . .

A psychiatric assessment could not find an easy diagnosis. She was not psychotic but her disturbed behaviour was extreme. She had some of the empty, repetitive behaviours of autistic children, but she was able to engage socially to a seemingly sophisticated level. The consultant psychiatrist commented on her poor attachment, her institutionalised quality of indiscriminate friendliness, and her production of stereotypes in artwork. Her classroom behaviour showed two extremes: excitedly barking, tearing at things and throwing things; then, by contrast, sucking her thumb and gazing into space for hours of time.

It remained a puzzle throughout Charlotte's therapy with me what exactly her diagnosis should be. Whilst therapy brought her genuine relief, containment, a measure of self-understanding, some reduction of anxiety and self-harm, it did not produce a normally developing young woman. Neither did her years accommodated in relatively benign residential institutions. Charlotte continued to exhibit her odd behaviours when under stress. Her learning remained limited and educationally she fell behind her peers year after year. It is therefore important to question in hindsight whether Charlotte's problems were likely to be accounted for by emotional or sexual abuse, even compounded as they were by neglect and physical abuse. Perhaps Charlotte's genetic endowment made her too vulnerable to experiences that scar and affect any child; perhaps there was early brain damage or inborn deficiency. Charlotte was examined by some of the best child mental health specialists of our time as her care was fiercely contested in a series of legal battles by her mother. Whilst the damage done to her by her abusive experiences was clear, the limited adjustment she made to life as a 'learning-disabled' adult indicated finally some developmental disorder however caused.

Charlotte's psychotherapy

I agreed to see Charlotte at the residential home where she lived and where I had a therapy room in one wing of the building. She visited me here three times every week.

Early themes in Charlotte's sessions revealed that she lived in an extremely primitive world. It is perhaps not surprising then that we spent a portion of almost every session in the toilet, which fortunately I had adjacent to my consulting room and within our private space. Although Charlotte often threatened to 'wee' or 'poo' on me and did wipe rather nasty body products on me once or twice, I could see that she was covering fear with bravado. I treated her as one would a young toddler, helping her, talking calmly about waste products coming out of the body, taking her manic excitement at the toilet flush as interest and letting her repeatedly pull the handle. I was, in effect, toilet training her. At the same time I contained her emotional turmoil and paid attention to the psychological significance of her worries, their meaning for her.

A blocked toilet

Charlotte strove to overcome her fear of her waste products by making someone else suffer them. This process can be referred to psychoanalytically as 'projective identification' (Ogden 1979: 357). She feared equally the toilet flush, the disappearance of what may be a part of her, and it transpired she feared a kind of retaliation from the toilet. Nevertheless she denied these fears with gusto and sought to inflict the fear on me. She relentlessly tried to block the toilet. Gradually I removed hand towels and other articles that could be thrown into the toilet bowl and doggedly restrained her from these escapades. I found I had one advantage in constraining her. She was, from the first, determined to have her sessions with me, so short removals because of uncontrollable behaviour were effective. She took seriously the threat of ending the session. I consistently offered to talk about her behaviour as a substitute for acting it out. We therefore had some interesting though peculiar conversations.

'I'm pooing too much today, ain't I? Will it all get blocked up? . . . I'll get off quick . . . It can go back up you, can't it?' These remarks revealed a girl who had no faith in there being a safe repository for waste products and whose idea of social relationships was retaliatory.

'If I break your doll's house you'll come to my room and break my stuff, won't you?' she had said on our first meeting. The experience of her sexual abuse was not mentioned in these early sessions but must have been around in her asking me in our sixteenth session: 'Inside me there's all these things, right, like in my mummy's tummy, where I came out of, right? Is there all those things in there as well? We went in a tortoise at the fair and it was all dark and smelly inside . . . if I went in your bottom it wouldn't be nice, would it? It would be all dark and smelly. My mum's coming tomorrow.'

As Melanie Klein pointed out, children think very concretely, and relate to the physicality of a mother's body (Klein 1975: 290). Charlotte seemed to be making a link between her own faeces, and the worry of getting rid of them, with herself coming from her mother's body. She did feel that she had been discarded into the children's home like a waste product. She felt she was like unwanted faeces. This was the way I tried initially to understand the confusion she poured into me. Charlotte felt herself to be a messed-up, messing baby in a contaminated world where there was little boundary between the baby and faeces. Inside the mother's body she imagined babies and poos in the same space – a dark smelly 'bottom world', as she began to express it to me.

I puzzled about the toilet being 'blocked' but at this time thought it must be about the absence of a mother who will clean the baby and separate her from the mess. Psychologically this would refer to the infant's understanding that a parent can cope with 'badness' and love the baby nonetheless. Without that she feared being flushed away herself.

Later, in her third year of therapy, this was more clearly expressed. She came into her session early in the morning and told me:

'I had a dream about my mummy. She was flushing a nappy out in the toilet, a baby's nappy and afterwards she washed her hands. But it was in the dirty water! Then I told her, "Stop! It's the smelly water!" She got so angry she tried to flush me down the toilet! Oh, I was covered with all poo and wee and all of that. And then she started sexing me and Grimlock [a character from TV] came in and pulled her off me and I was full of worms and wee and poo and a terrible smell – oh! oh!'

I interpreted this as Charlotte's fear that there would be no grown-up who could withstand mess or anger without retaliating. Charlotte's belief that adult sexuality is an exchange of faeces and her experience of sexual abuse widen her distrust of mother and of me. In transference terms it is I who attempt to clean up the baby. Charlotte fears my anger and sexuality. She fears what I will put into her.

Body boundaries, ego boundaries

It was characteristic of Charlotte that she had a poor sense of boundaries, both physical and psychological. In our fourth session she had told me she had a sore tongue and poked it out for me to see. 'Feel how sore it is,' she said, wanting me to touch it. She was insistent that I could feel its soreness by touching it. In later sessions she seemed to believe that I would actually feel her physical hurts in this way and it was not until the end of therapy, looking back with her, that I realised how deep and basic was this confusion. So, when I winced because she hit her head on the table she asked naively, 'Did you feel that?'

'No, but I imagined what it would feel like,' I replied.

'How can you do that?' she asked.

'Well, I think how I would feel if I hit my head.'

'Why?'

'I suppose it's automatic and because I care about you.'

'That's weird.'

I asked, 'Don't you ever imagine what I feel about something?'

'No,' was her innocent reply.

In fact this was so true that over the four years we met for therapy she never showed concern for any physical attack she made on me. When I was absent for illness she simply believed that I was tantalising or punishing her. I always made sure that I was well recovered after any absence as it would be followed by renewed attempts to bite or hit me.

Perhaps today Charlotte would be thought to have a developmental disorder such as Asperger's Syndrome (see Glossary). Her inability to empathise had severe repercussions for her relationships. She could not feel remorse or proper concern for others.

As a 7½-year-old in acute distress these features were not so noticeable nor as unusual as they later became. Children are more self-centred and empathy is expected to develop with maturity.

As her therapist, I continually marked out boundaries for Charlotte. I gradually and strenuously imposed order on our sessions. Without this it would have been impossible to withstand her physicality nor would there have been any thinking space for therapy. Charlotte learnt through consequences that she could not hurt me and continue with her session. She learned to substitute our discussions about insides and outsides and toilets and messes for her earlier attempts to inflict pain on me. Her willingness to come to her sessions and her reluctance to leave indicated that she found her therapy relieving. We were able to establish a 'talking and thinking space'. Nevertheless she continued to use 'whole-body' forms of play and was largely unable to use symbols or symbolic play. I functioned for her as an 'auxiliary' self and she remained limited in her ability to take in any identification with me.

Sexual abuse

I came to realise that when she talked about fairground rides, Charlotte was also alluding to her sexual abuse. The material was at first just suggestive and associative:

> We went in a tortoise at the fair and it was all dark and smelly inside . . . if I went in your bottom it wouldn't be nice would it? It would be all dark and smelly too. [Session 16]
>
> Shall we talk about the fair today? That wall ride where you stick to it, it's like wire, ain't it, and it goes round and round and it smells very awful, don't it . . . from all the smelly glue what makes it a sticking wall . . . and when you get off all that smelly glue – ugh . . . [Session 20]
>
> I'm on the spinning round and round ride! Mmm sex-y!

I tried initially to speak frankly to Charlotte about my understanding of the sexual details she was describing but this had eventually to be tempered by the knowledge that she used my words to gain further excitement. Gradually I learned to focus on her use of excitement to distract from pain and fear. She responded angrily to my sober responses, always seeking to provoke me into joining with her and claiming that I was excited too.

As we came up to a holiday break at Christmas, Charlotte's games became more noticeably about my absence and her abandonment. It was in this context that she told me in the fifth month of therapy that 'Bill' had taken her and her brother to the fairground. She told me this in a collected, calm manner and I thought she had thought consciously about revealing this to me. Then she told me she was making up a story about it in which she screamed at her brother, Eric, 'Don't go with him, he's dirty! Ugh, he's a smelly man! Throw the treats at him! Run away!' She told me briefly and seriously that Bill had 'sexed her' but 'she couldn't talk about it'. Eventually in this session she spun into her old routine of dizzying excitement and attack, ending our meeting in a frenzied attempt to pull apart an armchair and to bite me if I intervened.

In the following few sessions before Christmas it became apparent why Charlotte felt she could not appeal to her mother as a safe refuge against the abuser. She vividly enacted mother's intercourse with this boyfriend. The details were unmistakably accurate and she portrayed female orgasm as convincingly as she did male ejaculation. Her understanding of mother's intercourse was that it was anal, like her abuse.

In another session she graphically enacted a boyfriend 'going down the sewer to clear a blocked drain'. The 'sewer' was a blanket under which she writhed about suggestively.

In the context of our relationship in therapy I thought about why all these memories of mum and boyfriend were being brought up just before our Christmas holiday. Charlotte was perhaps assuming that I was abandoning her for my own sexual partner and that this was the meaning of our holiday break. Each session of our last fortnight ended in attacks on me when her 'enactments' got out of control. Finally, though, on our last session before Christmas she begged me at the end of our time to 'carry her out of her session like a baby'. Despite the risk of a nasty bite, I complied and she was the stiff corpse-like baby of the cliff. As I put her gently down at the door, she walked off, soberly, for once.

Piecing together these strands, which were worked over many times subsequently in her therapy, I became aware of a child who felt that she was stuck, that her mind was continually 'in her bottom', that she was both victim to a 'smelly man' and rival to her mother's union with a 'smelly man'. So Charlotte floundered in a 'sewer' in her mind where she could find no safe protective parent to clean her up and keep her in a child's position. As sexual partner to her mother's boyfriend she felt equated with her mother. Her child's view of sexuality was dominated by toilet imagery. Her emotional view of sexuality was contaminated with the fear and duress she had been put under by the perpetrator. She thought sexual intercourse was victimhood, a forced penetrative abuse of power over the frightened and powerless. The abuser's sexual excitement quelled the child's expression of fear. In her turn, Charlotte used excitement like a drug to numb any sense of her own pain or fear. Her hysterical, laughing, vengeful attacks on me could be understood as furious attacks on the 'sexual mother': she did indeed often grab my breast or my long hair. It was at times as if she was saying, 'Oh, you like this, do you? Well here it is!' What I was accused of liking was eroticised aggression, what Stoller (1986) called 'the erotic form of hatred'.

Freud deduced long ago that a child observing parental intercourse was inclined to see it as an aggressive act, a fight. Today we speculate that this would be because children are left out, angry and upset at the display of intimacy which they cannot comprehend. Klein emphasised the pain of exclusion felt by children when they realised they were not mother or father's partner. But a child with Charlotte's experience has additional reasons to fear parental intercourse. In her experience it is known to be aggressive and painful. Charlotte did not, however, consistently see her mother as a victim, but often as a co-perpetrator. This may have been due to the already poor relationship between them, her anger at mother's abandonment and her disbelief in mother's love. It may have been, as she occasionally claimed, that mother knew of and condoned Charlotte's sexual abuse. Mother's evident lack of boundary had the little girl in bed with her partner and herself during intercourse. I remained unsure about the extent of this involvement. Charlotte may have intruded into sexual scenes and mother may have been careless, disinhibited by drink, according to some of Charlotte's enactments. 'Bill' had also attacked mother, broken down their front door on one occasion as witnessed by a terrified Charlotte who repeated the details to me. He then got into bed with mother, according to Charlotte's traumatic, enacted 'flashbacks'. Without recourse to what Winnicott (1965) called 'the secure base' of a mother's concern Charlotte could only flee internally from these traumas. In therapy we attempted, so late in the day, to provide her with a place safe enough and a person available enough to begin to process these disturbing events.

The sinking mud of despair

One graphic and often-played-out idea of Charlotte's was that of quicksand or what she called 'the sinking mud'. In this story Charlotte plays the part of a lost animal who is sought and found by me. She tells me I am to 'find the baby cat stuck in the mud'. I am to come up to it and begin to pull it out. Only then am I to realise that this is 'sinking mud' and, if I don't get myself out and away, I will be pulled under by it. Charlotte's version of the story leaves no room for happier outcomes. Either I go under myself in this mud or I escape and leave the baby to drown.

We talked about this game on several occasions. I think its main import related to Charlotte's despair that there could be a rescuer strong enough to save the baby as well as herself. In this version of mothering the mother needs to be heroic and strong but is doomed to failure. There is no notion of a 'parental couple' or cooperative mutually supporting adults who act in concert to care for a child. It has to be said that Charlotte's experience of her own mother mitigated against this idea. But also, Charlotte's possessiveness, omnipotence and rage left her stranded in helplessness. These 'sinking mud' games often followed any holidays I had from her. She did not believe that I could hold onto her emotionally nor she onto me during these separations. Her version of my holidays was always one of my abandonment.

At least in these stories Charlotte began partly to identify herself with someone who needed rescue, who was in need of help. A number of games then followed on this theme of failed rescue. I shall quote extensively from one which followed my six-week summer holiday after two years of therapy.

The session begins with her asking me to play hide-and-seek. When I find her she tells me, 'I'm not Charlotte, I'm a little cat. But I've seen Charlotte, she's with the smelly man! He's getting her drunk, giving her beer and lager and now he's cuddling her . . . he's doing bad wrestling to her – she's almost bleeding . . . call the police.' Charlotte now switches her role and pretends that she is the police.

The police spend all their time chasing the 'smelly man' and then enacting a crucifixion of him: 'Knock those sharp nails right through his hands, serves him right.' I point out that no one in the story seems to be caring how Charlotte is or making sure she feels better. Charlotte responds by telling me she becomes a cat in the story and is given to a man to be looked after. At first this man is kind but he turns into Superman and now it's 'the bad Superman because he's getting a suntan in a brown submarine. There are two of them who look the same . . . F—— off, Mrs Hunter!' She rushes into my bathroom and throws the toilet roll into the toilet bowl.

My interpretation of the story is as follows. Charlotte feels the need to be found and to have me look for her and find her. Hide-and-seek is one of a child's earliest attachment games, re-enacting under her own control the experience of loss and recovery of mother's absence and return. The recent experience here is the summer holiday. Charlotte, now aged 9, behaves like a delighted younger child as she waits for me to find her, to repair my abandonment of her between sessions and in the holiday.

Her game moves into another dimension when she tells me that I am not able to reach her because she is in the control of the sexual abuser, the 'smelly man'. She believes I must rescue her from this position.

As well as a re-enactment of the past. I believe the 'smelly man' stands for my husband in the transference. Charlotte's association with him is her rivalry with me in my assumed sexual preoccupation.

When I and the forces of authority, the police, do find Charlotte in her game, vengeance takes over so strongly that the hurt child is overlooked. I intervene to point this out. Charlotte's reply is that she has become a cat with daddy/Superman who cannot be trusted because he looks identical to a sexually preoccupied male. I think this is the meaning of a Superman getting a suntan. The 'brown submarine' has phallic and faecal connotations.

This would mean that Charlotte's belief in my power to rescue her is obstructed. My absence in the holidays seems to mean to her that she is left with a sexual male who is getting a 'suntan' and is suspiciously like an abuser. Furiously she blocks up my toilet to show me she is still where she began, unable to flush away contaminating badness, still stuck in the toilet, her mind in her bottom. Charlotte's incapacity to hold onto an identification with a hurt child is also clear in this story. She manages it for a short period whilst I am made to actively look for her. But the need for revenge on me, the need to rival me, the graphic wish to hurt and maim a sexual partner and her escape into excitement, attack and destructive power is all too clear. Thus she ends up attacking me, blocking my toilet and telling me in aggressive sexual terms to 'F—— off!' She is at this point in identification with the abuser.

For many months following, Charlotte's games worked and reworked the theme of how a child can relate to a mother when the mother has a relationship with a man. This material was related to Charlotte's real-life experiences but it was also Oedipal in the way that Freud observed (see Glossary). The child's jealousy and possessiveness of the mother makes her view the parental couple with suspicion, with anger, with fear. Melanie Klein further emphasised the child's wish to attack and destroy the couple, in her rage at being excluded.

Jaws: the biting baby

It seemed to me that I had to wrestle again and again with Charlotte's infatuation with a fantasy of excitement and power that kept her enthralled and unable to relate properly to me or anyone else. In her fantasy, she was savage and powerful, able to inflict hurt, able to be an aggressor rather than a victim.

I often puzzled at the strength and vehemence of this illusion. I reasoned that it could not just have appeared when she was 5, despite my appreciation of the horror of her abuse. Then I began to disentangle earlier ideas that related to her earlier relationship with her mother and to focus on these.

In her first year of therapy Charlotte had begun in a calm manner to tell me that she had been allowed to watch the film *Jaws*. To my surprise as she began to explain the plot her lip trembled and she began to sob piteously: one of the few occasions when I saw her show genuine grief.

'They tricked him,' she sobbed. 'He thought it was something to eat but it was all wees and poos and bad food poison and when he bit it, it was a bomb. He got exploded into pieces.'

The whole session was taken up with her asking me whether it was right to blow up the shark. He had been biting and hurting people. He bit the food and it killed him. 'Would you kill that shark?' she asked anxiously.

In this way I understood that Charlotte felt identified with this fierce, biting, destructive creature. She feared her own extinction in a retaliatory world. She needed to believe that I was compassionate enough to save a shark like herself.

However, we heard no more of Jaws for a long time. What we did hear about was a cheeky cartoon character, 'Woody Woodpecker'. This character first appeared several months after 'Jaws', in the following way.

She asked me to find her in a game of hide-and-seek. When I do, I am told 'It's Woody Woodpecker! You take him home with you.'

'What would happen then?' I ask.

'When you wake up in the morning all the house is eaten up and Woody Woodpecker is snoring! He's eaten everything! All the food, all the chairs and table, all the cups and saucers. You buy a new house for a hundred pounds.'

Charlotte explains that I keep buying new houses and she, as Woody Woodpecker, gets up in the night and voraciously devours everything in sight. Finally I want to get rid of Woody and I get it 'put down'. But I am to buy a new one 'who is very good by trying hard'. Gradually he resumes his old ways and starts eating everything up . . . he is stuffed into the dustbin . . . then he is stuffed 'between the smelly man's legs'. I am told to chase the smelly man with a carving knife . . . the Woody Woodpecker character gets forgotten as chases and fights between the 'mother' and the 'smelly man' take over the action.

My understanding of this and similar games is that Charlotte identified herself with a voraciously hungry, destructive baby 'Woody'. In the role play of exasperated mother and a creature who literally eats them out of house and home, 'Woody' brings a series of reprisals on himself, including being rubbished and being 'stuffed' into a sexually abusive situation. The mother is depicted as provoked, then exasperated, then abandoning, then revengeful, in turn. I think this is Charlotte's understanding of her own mother's attitude toward her. It was also Charlotte's understanding of herself as an impossibly greedy child. Charlotte believed there was a rough justice in her abandonment and her sexual abuse.

Talking with Charlotte about her belief that she was a greedy baby who feared she deserved abandonment and abuse did seem to bring her relief and a degree of understanding. After several reworkings of the Woody Woodpecker story in which she desperately tried to reconcile the mother and this cheeky, greedy character she made up a game where the mother is dying. At this point she dropped 'Woody' and made me be the one who goes to my home to find mother dead. Charlotte burst into real tears whilst I stopped playing and talked gently about her fear of losing her mother, of her fear that she deserves abandonment, because of her destructiveness.

The parental couple

It seemed after a year and a half of therapy that Charlotte may have been coming to terms with her idea of herself as a powerfully destructive child in a retaliatory relationship. Therapy was experienced at last as a non-retaliatory relationship where I could withstand her hatred and aggression. But the necessary sequestration of a mother–infant relationship seemed to last only fleetingly. There was scarcely any peace between us of this kind. Instead there was presented, with soul-destroying repetitiveness for me, the constant theme of sexual excitement interrupting the possibility of mother–child exchanges.

The infantile part of Charlotte never could find enduring peace in the arms of a mother because the mother's relationship to a sexual and brutal male always intervened. This was her experience of her own mother and continued to be how Charlotte interpreted all my holiday breaks from her therapy. She felt I abandoned her for my sexual partner. This man would not be a 'daddy' but a competitor for my affection. Faced with the prospect of being left out whilst the 'parental couple' were together in bed Charlotte desperately tried to make herself the 'provider' (as Woody Woodpecker reformed). But her hunger and anger and wish to be powerful produces bad food. Charlotte cannot allow mother to be restored by someone else. Charlotte internally allies herself with the sexual abuser in a triumphant competitive stance against my imagined sexual union.

I puzzled very often how to get Charlotte out of this deadlock where she endlessly invited abuse as a spiteful retaliation to the version of me she felt was real. I found it hard to understand how relentlessly repetitive the material still was and how little it gave way to interpretation, how little it changed despite our relationship and the trust she had built up in me. It was three months after this that it was discovered that a teenage boy in the home was sexually abusing her.

Sexual abuse in a community home

It was tempting to believe that Charlotte invited her abuse and gained satisfaction from outwitting me and competing with me. Remembering that she was 10 years of age at this time and discovering that several children were abused and bullied by this boy, it is clearer that she was also afraid and bullied into compliance. But most of her sessions during this time were filled with triumphalism whereas the despair was felt by me, split off into me. The mind can tell itself protective stories and Charlotte's was one of identification with a selfish, aggressively sexual therapist. Perhaps too, it recreated too nearly her original abuse, under her mother's nose, so to speak and during her mother's absence.

Here is a session from the time period when she was, unknown to me, being sexually abused again:

> Charlotte begins the session with the 'sinking mud' and tells me that I am to watch her drown. I talk about her despair, her belief I cannot help without endangering myself, her belief in our equality, that I am no stronger than her.
>
> She changes her story. 'A boy called Keith is down the sewer fixing a pipe. There are wees and poos and all that and you want to go in too. He's banging a lot.' 'Why would I want to go down?' I ask. 'Oh, stop gabbing on! I'll do it myself. You've got to be quiet – but you see a tunnel and you say "I wonder what's down there?",' she instructs me. 'We seem to be in a bottom place . . . there's a child who's very curious and left out and wants to get into a place she shouldn't be,' I say.
>
> Charlotte is annoyed and tells me to 'shut up'. Impatiently she makes up a game without me. She pretends to make a circle with other 'Transformers' and they dance around 'creating a new Autobot'. I try to discuss whether this is a creation story to get rid of mothers and fathers or to dispense with her idea of me and a boyfriend. She asks plaintively if I will play hide-and-seek. When I shut my eyes she urinates in my cupboard . . .

I see the meaning of this session as Charlotte descending into her bottom world with her own 'boyfriend'. She imagines herself in the same sexual/toilet world that she thinks I inhabit without her and where she is forbidden. Disrupted by my attempts to discuss this she plays out another version of her rivalry with me: in this the children create a baby between themselves. Again interrupted, she asks me to play the game which symbolises our separation, hide-and-seek. Instead of being reparative and reciprocal she tricks me and wees in my cupboard. My trust is betrayed with an angry infantile attack. On another level one could say she imagines she gets inside me and messes me up inside, weeing in me. Or that sexual intercourse is portrayed as urinating inside a forbidden place. Her sexual abuse by the teenager does fulfil a function in satisfying her curiosity and envy of me.

The struggle to shut the bedroom door

Working with Charlotte, three days a week, forty-six weeks a year for four years, I look back now with amazement at the power of her delusion and with despair that she could ever leave her perverse world. She buoyed herself up on a hysterical wave of excitement and aggression. Her belief in her culpability and her abandonment to fight and flight, mitigated against her gaining control over her addiction to excitement.

One particular difficulty for Charlotte was the unstable nature of any good figure in her mind. So a kind character could, without warning, become bad and attacking. She herself could find no equilibrium and was beset by her rages, at the mercy of her emotional tides. Gradually she perceived that I and others had more control, but mainly she believed this was the cleverness of my deception. She could not believe consistently in anyone.

However, we did together come to a greater understanding and a greater sense of mastery over the demons that ruled her. She began to see for herself that she needed to control her fierce greed and curiosity. Here is a session from her third year of therapy. At this point she was finally able to use symbolic play in the form of small Playmobil dolls.

> She set up a game where a mother and father take a baby to the park. They leave the baby on a swing saying, 'Don't swing too high', and they go away. When they return the baby is swinging too high and they shout at the 'playground lady' and at the baby.
>
> We discuss this, with my emphasising that it is parents who must guard and keep the baby safe. The baby is left and fills up the

> emptiness with excitement, not really understanding the danger. She plays that the mother and father take the baby home. They begin to kiss and cuddle each other but the mum says, 'Oh, not in front of her, remember, it's not good for her.' They place the baby 'in her own bed'. They begin to 'make love'. The baby cries and asks to join in. 'No.' The door is shut. The baby goes to sleep. There is a long sequence of Charlotte making the mother and father dolls have sex.

In this session we see Charlotte struggling with ideas of a baby who is neglected and gets into danger. This develops into a discussion with me about responsibility and the need for a baby to be protected. Her play then incorporates this idea with the baby left out of the parents' sexual intercourse, not from neglect, but for her own protection. The parents' bedroom door seems finally able to be shut. But Charlotte finds identification with the sleeping baby hard to maintain and continues in her fantasy to be preoccupied with the parental intercourse.

Nevertheless there was a containment to these sessions which was markedly absent from the earlier years. The breakthrough into symbolic play was an immense achievement because it allowed different emotional positions (i.e. the baby, the mother and father) to be explored simultaneously. This happened within a framework where Charlotte was the storyteller or puppet master so that there was less of her becoming lost in the excitement of acting out a role with her whole body. She and I could be onlookers to the drama.

In a similar vein, this session from the end of the third year finds Charlotte preparing to move on:

> She tells me the figures are 'Transformer' robots and lines them up in pairs. One is 'Master Motor' and is placed a little apart. The pairs of robots start 'snogging and kissing and all that', she tells me. She makes them writhe about together. 'Master Motor' is leaving home and kisses all of them goodbye. There is a moment when 'Master Motor' hesitates and wants to become a couple with one of the robots but he decides its better to have his own base . . .
>
> She takes six sheets of paper, counting them out for the sides, top and bottom of a house. Despite their flimsiness she succeeds in gluing together four walls and a floor. She cuts out a door and windows. At several points she has to struggle with the paper threatening to collapse and her impulse to pull it apart. We talk about the frustration of trying to make something and how easy it would be to join in with

> the forces of destruction. . . . [In the following session she continued and completed the 'base'.]

In this way Charlotte tentatively turned herself toward creativity and hopefulness. Her sexual preoccupations clearly continued to hold fascination for her but there was, at last, a wish to bracket off sexual excitement from other interests. Making a house, albeit one in which she was alone and still an over-powerful figure, 'Master Motor', was an acknowledgement of her need for security and protection. The idea of having a 'base' contrasts forcefully with her repetitive drowning in the 'sinking mud'. With this degree of fragile integration Charlotte aged 11 took her leave from me, moving to a small therapeutic community.

Chapter 6

Child sexual abuse

Defence mechanisms

- placation and denial
- a legacy of lies
- the role of power and control
- counter-transference experiences
- projective identification in abuse
- bullying
- rules and boundaries
- borderline personality disorder
- dissociation and splitting
- false memory
- self-abuse

Charlotte's story in the preceding chapter is one of sexual abuse happening very early in a child's developing life. Her development was already awry, with poor attachment to her mother, no 'secure base' as Winnicott called it, little belief in a mother's protection or availability for help. So Charlotte buoyed herself up with an illusion that distracted her from her perilous and helpless position. She became addicted to excitement and mania, employing aggression and sexuality to give the chimera of power and virility. Perhaps this is the key to the sexually abusive personality, the characteristics of a perpetrator. We know from recent research (Farmer and Pollock 1998; Hodges *et al.* 1997: 120) that a proportion of sexually abused children will go on to become perpetrators, whilst others will continue to present themselves as ready victims. Charlotte's encounter with an older boy in the children's home had perhaps both aspects of this legacy.

Of the eighty children in care who joined me in therapy and who are principally the subjects of this book, thirty-two had been sexually abused. This high proportion reflects the high number of children accommodated following sexual abuse in childhood. Research evidence indicates that the effects of sexual abuse on youngsters are far-reaching. Low self-esteem, self-injurious behaviour, depression, post-traumatic stress syndrome and an increased risk of adult mental illness are associated outcomes (Farmer and Pollock 1998; Mrazek and Kempe 1987).

These research findings derive from quantitative surveys where the links between antecedent conditions and outcomes are beginning to be established. The value of working closely, intimately, with thirty-two looked-after children who have experienced sexual abuse is that one gets to understand the how and the why of the harm done to these children. The themes that I can identify in my work with them are those with which I have found myself wrestling as we have inched our way back to non-abusive relationships.

More pervasive and more troubling than the physical trauma is the web of deception and manipulation into which these children fall. A world where you cannot trust, where weakness is exploited, where dependence is betrayed, is a truly nightmarish existence. I therefore perceive the severity of sexual abuse not in terms of, for example, penetrative versus non-penetrative sexuality, nor even violent or non-violent abuse. I conceptualise sexual abuse primarily in relationship terms. If the abuser was a parent on whom the child had to depend, then relationships which should involve protection and dependency will be affected. If the abuse was secretive, manipulative, involving the child for months or years as a participant, then these facets will permeate the child's relationships to all others. In hostage situations it is common to identify with the perpetrator in order to keep safe and many sexually abused children do so. Hostages monitor their kidnappers minutely in order to anticipate and placate them. Conflict can mean pain or even death, so it is avoided assiduously.

The younger the child the greater is the degree of dependence and the more development will have to take place around and through the abuse. Where a young child grows up being sexually abused in the first few years of life they seem to suffer the worst consequences to their character. Some can scarcely reflect, identify their own feelings and have awareness of their own worth. These children seem in a constant state of hyper-vigilance and their relationships seem dominated by fight or flight (see Jody in Chapter 9). There can even be an absence of trauma as we identify it because the child has insufficient sense of self to protest, to feel 'wounded'. If all of life is unsafe the capacity for shock or protest dies out: placatory flatness is left. Where the child is already a functioning and relatively sound individual, sexual abuse does constitute an assault on the self and the young person will protest with pain and exhibit symptoms.

Lying and truth

A child can be sexually abused by someone they don't know who has little connection with their lives. If their relationship to a parent is secure enough and they have access to that parent, they can tell, the parent will intervene and the abuse will stop. Such a child will have experienced a trauma, an assault on their body and on their sense of self. But they will have also experienced their protected status, their worth to the parent, and their right to inviolability. Children in the care system are rarely of this group. What characterises children protected by Care Orders is usually the lack of an adequate parent. Thus the child may not tell or may tell and not be believed or be believed but not protected. Compounding the assault on their body is the implication that they have no access to and no right to protection. If the external world does not adequately protect, the internal world must do so. Thus a range of defence mechanisms, denial, dissociation, fantasy will be employed to protect the self from terror and despair. The lies that we tell ourselves are often functional lies, meant to protect us from knowing what we cannot bear. Abused children commonly therefore have to resort to self-protective lies. This is one raft of untruths.

Child sexual abusers have to keep their victims quiet. Threats of harm if the child tells are therefore usual. The child must be prevailed upon to lie, to cover up the abusive experiences or, at minimum, to keep quiet about it. The threats, fear of discovery and fear of harm account for a second raft of untruths.

If the child lives with the abuser, day after day, minute by minute, lies run through the relationship that the child must appear to have with the abuser. Living with an abusive father or stepfather means that the whole appearance of family life is a dissemblance, a charade for any observers who do not know the truth. If the mother is one of these observers then the child's relationship to her is affected: the child has to be cautious and non-spontaneous or the truth may be blurted out. If the mother knows, perhaps she lies about it to herself and pretends it is not happening or that it is not significant. Parents who have themselves been sexually abused, who employed protective self-deceptions and lived in situations where little was what it seemed, more easily repeat the failure to protect which happened to them.

One young adolescent, Ashley, asked me for help in telling her mother that grandad had sexually molested her. We met together several times and when her daughter's abuse was finally undeniable the mother said that she was also sexually abused as a child, but she didn't go around stealing like Ashley, she just got on with life. Why didn't Ashley?

Ashley's mother could not act as a protective parent because she had convinced herself as a child that there were no protective parents.

But most insidious of all is a powerful raft of lies that most sexual abusers have to employ in order to abuse. These lies are concerned with denying the fear and misery of the child and substituting the abuser's own sexual excitement and sense of power. Abusers do not take in the fear of their victim except to dismiss or denigrate these emotions. Abusers employ sexual excitement as a mask and distraction to the real interchange between themselves and the victim. In this way there is an assault on the victim's truth, on the victim's reality. Children are told that they do not feel what they feel, that the abuser's reality is what counts. One important aspect of this is what happens to the victim's sense of reality and truth. I meet children who have been so systematically abused that to them truth is whatever the most powerful person says it is. What is real is the other and they expect to have little say in that.

Thus the very basis of interaction between themselves and others is undermined in these abused children. They believe that they have no personal claim on truth or reality.

A girl of 12, Blossom, was referred to me following the disclosure of regular sexual abuse from the age of 7. She agreed that the man had sexual intercourse with her, that it hurt, that she tried to avoid it and was pleased when he did not pick her up from school. He was her older sister's partner. But she did not want him prosecuted, seemed not to understand what the fuss was about or why he should be punished. In her therapy it emerged that he had systematically quelled any sign of protest from her. She became used to obedience and compliance as the quickest way to get the experiences over. Gradually she 'forgot' that there was any sense of non-compliance on her part and went along with his definition of the situation. Having put away her own sense of outrage she was like an automaton, blank, passive, acquiescent. Her feelings were reduced to insignificant whispers that she assumed everyone, including herself, should ignore.

Trust, mistrust and betrayal

Charlotte, in the preceding chapter, played games where a family picnicked with a 'kind brown bear'. It suddenly erupted into a violent attack when its 'long brown fur' was stroked. The bear then attacked and terrorised everyone. It returned to being 'nice' with no guarantee whatsoever that it would not suddenly flare up again. Thus, in subsequent sessions, the brown bear, however kind it was being in her game, could not be trusted. It was truly maddening to be urged to enjoy myself and to be silenced by her excitedly shouting over me if I voiced concerns. As if the abuser were really in the room with us, she once whispered to me, 'Watch out, you're gonna really get it now for saying that.' Charlotte believed that the truth must not be spoken and must be forgotten.

The fourth raft of lies that I have had to define in order to try to recover such children involves the abuser's pleasure in the power of lies. I found Wilfred Bion's writing of help here:

> Some forms of lying appear to be closely related to experiencing desire. Long stories with every appearance of truth are spun out extempore as if the virtuosity of the exercise gave pleasure . . . For satisfaction the liar needs an audience . . . The thinker is logically necessary for the lie . . . The thinker is of no consequence to the truth.
>
> (Bion 1971: 104)

This extract makes evident the sense of power and control that is inherent in a lie. Liars can feel that they create their own universe. If they can make others believe in their fabrications it can be felt as a sense of secret control over others.

Nathan: trapped in lies

Nathan, a teenage boy of 13 years, was befriended by a paedophile who enmeshed him in a web of lies. Nathan's parents had split up after months of acrimony. Whilst they were involved in their arguments and access battles they did not at first notice Nathan's absence as he more and more called at the nearby flat of his friend. This friend seemed nothing but kindness to the unhappy boy, even letting Nathan share his beer. He constantly told him what a great boy he was. As Nathan began to get uncomfortable with the way the friendship was developing and began to withdraw this man 'revealed' that he had a terminal illness. The compassionate boy began to get the man's prescriptions and shopping and to feel that he could not abandon his friend. Eventually, and by degrees, the man raped Nathan. The boy had enough self-respect not to return to the man's flat but this was not the end of the matter. The abuser constantly followed and harangued Nathan with stories of his ill health. Finally, Nathan's mother took out an injunction against the man's harassment, not knowing of the sexual abuse. The family began to receive phone calls from this man's son who claimed to be depressed about his father's illness. Receiving a call that this son had taken an overdose, Nathan's mother involved the police in a search for this suicidal young man who was not found. Soon after this the police established the abuser's rape of several other children and Nathan confessed his own sexual abuse. In the police investigations that followed, it transpired that the abuser had no illness and no son. Using an assumed voice the abuser himself had played out the whole charade of a suicidal 'son' over the phone.

In Nathan's therapy he was perhaps as harmed and confused by the lies as he was by the rape. At least in the rape he felt he had a moment of clarity when he knew that he was being badly used. As he had struggled with the manipulations of this paedophile, his guilt at not caring for a 'sick kind man' had really haunted him. Now looking back he was in despair. He was filled with embarrassment and hated his trusting self. He despised his own kindness and naivety and he spoke bitterly of himself and his trustfulness. It took many meetings to try to ease Nathan's self-condemnation and put it where it belonged. Embarrassment is a powerful and much underrated emotion. Shame at being gullible is powerfully felt by child victims.

Power and control

The web of lies with which an abuser manipulates a child is not incidental, it is an integral part of the event. The victim is left to struggle with incompatible emotions that will not fit together. Sexually abusive adults can believe that they like children, and be kind to children. They are available, they tell the child they are special. Split off, away from consciousness, there is the attack and the manipulation of the child until the point of force. The abuser routinely ignores this reality. The child victim is bewildered by the range of emotions displayed, by the excitement of the abuser, by the confused jumble of messages. The abuser ignores the child's expressions of fear and intimidation. Children feel they cannot have shouted loudly enough or plainly enough. Faced with a more powerful adult who imposes their view of what is happening onto scared children, these children often give up their own view, feeling they must be incorrect, they must be wrong.

I have understood this from what older children can put into words but I know it most often from the frightening feelings that I have had pushed into me from these children, in what is called the 'counter-transference' (see Glossary).

The counter-transference of many sexually abused children is one where I experience bewilderment and compliance. These children seize power in my room, they bombard me with commands, with diversions, with urgent passionate demands for me to comply. Finding myself taken aback, semi-compliant, bewildered, uncomprehending, it may only be later that I realise how exactly an experience of abuse has been lodged in me. A therapist stands before a patient with willingness to receive, to listen, to meet them more than halfway. An abused patient who is driven by the compulsion to abuse will ride roughshod over protests, attempts to think or slow down, will drown out the voice of reason, of thoughtfulness. This experience will closely mirror the abusive experience. With children like Charlotte one may be confronted with a blocked or overflowing faecal mess which puts the counter-transference into very concrete terms. With another child, 7-year-old Zoe, her bombardment of me used to culminate in her somehow getting into a position where she was lying on the floor and I was standing astride her. These experiences amplify those which are more subtle. The confusion engendered by being harangued and bullied or charmed and seduced by such children is a counter-transference confusion. As an inexperienced therapist I used to mistake it for my own inability, just like my patients who mistake their confusion as belonging to and originating in themselves. They think that their sexual abuse is their own embarrassment, their own shame. It is the abuser's shame that they have incorporated. 'Projective identification' is a psychoanalytic term used to describe a phenomenon that can happen between two people whereby one person pushes an unwanted feeling into the other and then acts as if it belongs to that person (projection), leaving the other to feel identified with this projection. Both parties can then act as if the unwanted feeling were really part of the recipient rather than the originator.

In psychotherapy it is possible, finally, within a transference relationship (see Glossary), to address who is responsible for which feelings and to observe and understand the way feelings can flow back and forth between two people.

Zoe: abuse is better than abandonment

Nathan told me that at least he understood that he was being attacked when he was raped. Some children who are seduced remain confounded by the nature of the action done to them. Zoe, at 7 years, maintained that sex was 'good' and that she had enjoyed it. She shocked staff in her children's home by loudly proclaiming that she wanted 'someone to sex her tonight'. In her highly charged sessions with me, she fought to have control. She made a paper set of keys with which to let herself in and out of my consulting room. Telling me 'go to bed, it's night-time', she pulled the curtains, darkened the room and locked the door. I was to be all alone listening to noises and to wonder if I was being left alone 'for ever'. I was to have no keys. When a man came, at last, it was clear that there would be a mixture of relief and fear in the encounter. She would roll up some 'ganja' and make a chicken supper. Only, somehow, I would get pinched or have the food fall on me, or be pushed roughly, still being told how we were having 'a great time, eh?'. It was a lonely, unsatisfactory encounter where my bewilderment was ignored and the questions I asked were left unanswered. I had a very clear picture from this of Zoe's own experiences.

Children think very concretely. If someone gives them 'presents' they feel that person must be kind. If someone lets them share alcohol or drugs they feel privileged. The powerful can command even the language in which an event is described and thereby distort it. 'My uncle loves me and gives me lots of presents' or 'I'm daddy's special girl' can be words that distort and misrepresent the events they purport to describe. Often with sexually abused children I find I am trying to re-label and re-describe events that have hidden a lie. Human beings have fortunately an instinct for truth that is not easily or completely perverted. These children's scenarios of seduction are not happy and enjoyable. They invariably contain blows, hurts, pinches, aggression, threats. Words are often at variance with actions. No wonder such children watch me and my words so intently and refuse to be impressed by my linguistic skill. They fight for control of the session: they think that power is abused by adults. When they are in charge they are despotic, delinquent. They are also, it must be said, very good at seizing their opportunities. They have learned only too well the mechanisms of bullying.

Breaking boundaries

Abused children believe in power and rarely in authority. Their experiences have been that adults are self-seeking and control things for their own ends. In traumatic form it has been made plain to them that their body boundaries are not inviolable, that they are permeable, that forced entry is possible. This seems to give added dimension to the child's desire to seize power. Trust is not possible so control is substituted. Such children see all relationships as being between bullies and victims. If you are a liberal, gentle adult, many abused children will try to victimise you. Many such children will hurl themselves at any boundary or limit set for them, their actions flooded with the meaning 'rules are made for breaking'. These children gain great relief from the calm, contained enforcement of limits. By this means the therapist demonstrates, more effectively than any words can say, that she believes in limits, that boundaries will be respected, that the bully will not rule. It seems that the child may need to see this repetitively before they can begin to believe that the reign of terror is over. A child learns by example how to stand up to threat and intimidation without the endless recycling of it between bully and victim. Charlotte's plaintive 'If I broke your toys you'd come and break mine, wouldn't you?' expresses this relentless exchange. Not breaking Charlotte's toys, but firmly preventing her from breaking mine, gives her a hope that one can emerge from a cycle of retaliatory attack. Attacking boundaries can be a symbolic enactment of the child's despair. It can also contain their hope that someone will stop this travesty of order.

As well as the physical boundaries of the setting and the person of the therapist which can come under attack there are psychological boundaries which can be similarly threatened. Some children seem quite unclear where they end and you begin. Sexual and emotional abuse often has a causative link to this condition because the abuser has denied and distorted the boundary between themselves and the child. In the psychiatric condition known as 'borderline personality' (see Glossary) the adult patient seems continually to misrepresent where their own self and responsibility lie in relation to others. They fear separation and are intolerant of difference because a form of merger is essential to the way they operate psychologically: in effect they need the other person to carry unwanted parts of themselves. Many borderline adults have been abused children (Fonagy *et al.* 1995).

Children who are recipients of a powerful adult acting in this mode will become unclear about their own boundaries and borders. To be made to carry parts of the adult as if they were your own can result in the belief that the self is bad and responsible for these attributes. Furthermore, developing within this regime it may ultimately become necessary for the child to employ another person to carry all these unwanted, intolerable aspects that they cannot manage. Thus they are set up to repeat with their foster carer, their partner, or eventually their own child a similar interaction of misery.

Marilyn: is reality a dream?

A young woman who seemed to be poised at the brink of this kind of development was Marilyn. She seemed when I first met her to be floating through her life in a fog of little feeling. She reported an inability to be alone, needing to be accompanied for any journey, and she was unable to feel all right in a room on her own. She thought that when others looked at her they would see her as odd. Actually she was rather beautiful.

Marilyn was a tall, well-developed girl who looked much older than 15. She had been placed in a secure unit following a string of offences for theft and an alarming series of near-death drug experiences. She had a dreamy, vacuous air and a sweet smile. She smiled when describing her overdoses and seemed unperturbed by her experiences although she would admit to preferring life outside of a secure unit. I saw her when she had been transferred to specialist foster care. In therapy sessions she gradually let me know that her older brother had forced Marilyn to have sex with him when she was 11. After some months of putting up with this she told her mother. Her mother beat her brother, chasing him through the house in a loud fury, hitting him with a belt. He still forced her to have sex with him after this beating but as she grew older she became more adept at avoiding him and he gradually stopped. However, when she had revealed this unhappy story to a social worker her mother denied the story adamantly. Her brother also denied it. Ejected from the family she went on wild drug binges to bombard her anxieties into submission. As months elapsed she realised that having any relationship with her family depended on her giving up her account of past events. She tried therefore to give up her memories. 'Perhaps it was a dream,' she said to me. 'I don't really know it happened. If they're sure it didn't happen, maybe I dreamt it.' I took seriously the proposition that her memory was faulty and at various times we would look at her capacity for knowing reality from fantasy.

My first impression of Marilyn would have been consistent with her not having a strong sense of reality. However, despite her dreamy air, she gave internally consistent and coherent accounts of present happenings and past events. Her brother's beating on the former occasion was only one in a series of regular assaults her mother made on them both. She told me quite coolly how regularly and brutally she was beaten by her mother. The hardest part she told me was to learn 'not to put up your arms' to defend yourself. That brought a further fury of blows from mum. 'You had to keep still and take it. Then it would be over quicker.' In this cruel regime she had already learned to suffer quietly. There was the added complication that she and her brother were both victims and a certain amount of alliance against their mother was present. There was no sense in which his advances had been welcome or comforting, however. According to her account he seemed instead to be depositing his anger at his mother's assaults into her. In a home where she was the victim of assault from two directions she tried hard to avoid conflict, to placate, to smile and to make her defences unnoticeable. Drugs seemed to offer a way to get 'out of her head' and to change the only thing she could: herself. But under the influence of drugs her anger and despair broke loose and she always went over the top, pursuing death as a solution to her pain.

With her dreamy, switched-off look and her wish to blur her sense of reality, Marilyn was on the path to disabling herself. If she takes sufficient drugs over a sufficient amount of time perhaps she will lose her grasp of what has or has not happened to her. She may be able to become culpable for the awfulness of her life.

Listening to her I became aware of the unbearable position of being a helpless beaten child who knows she does not deserve her treatment. The pain of knowing this was such that she could prefer to destroy her own apparatus for knowing her own mind. Alternatively she could become someone who deserved abuse. She could become her own abuser and have some power over her fate.

Dissociation and false memory

Despite Marilyn's attempts to lose consciousness of events she could not bear, she was able to talk about them with coherence. It has been my experience that traumatic events like sexual abuse cannot be easily shut out of consciousness. The power of the event is sometimes so strong that victims do not want to discuss the details or find that they are wary of triggering the emotions of which the facts are part. Some victims feel it is like re-experiencing the abuse if they think too much about it. Ordinary processes of diversion, distraction and avoidance can be used to avoid these painful memories.

Sometimes victims can present the facts of their abuse but their emotions are clearly elsewhere. They have effected a split between the event and its associated misery. This split state was illustrated by Marilyn's casual account of her heart stopping in the ambulance on her way to casualty. No mention was made of a sense of danger or concern that the event should have triggered. When a person presents painful or traumatic events with a marked absence of emotion or inappropriate emotion, it is rightly called 'dissociated'. Of course, it is possible to mistake the significance of dissociation or to identify it wrongly. A victim who has given several accounts of an event may find the emotional aspects of it subside. Time and integration of an event make it less 'raw'. We do not call people 'dissociated' because they can talk equably of a death several years ago, though we might if the death was days ago. Dissociation is therefore an internal psychological state which we assume is present when a usual or expected involvement of emotion is absent. The counter-transference feeling to a dissociated patient can be one of absence and remove from the patient: but often the therapist may feel that they are flooded with emotion whilst the patient seems to have none. I keenly remember Marilyn's advice to me 'not to put up your arms' if you are being hit.

Alison's wonderful parents

I treated for three years a young woman, Alison, who had been unspeakably sexually and emotionally abused by her parents. She could not easily bring these memories to discuss because she felt flooded with despair and pain which was difficult for her to manage when the session ended. I learnt to help her contain this misery by addressing small pieces of it at a time and making sure that we ended each session firmly in the present, not in the midst of past memories. Despite the horror of her life she seemed to have access to these memories at will. She described, however, many defensive mechanisms of keeping herself busy or distracted to stop the memories intruding. She suffered from 'flashbacks' (see Glossary), unwanted intrusive thoughts about her experiences of rape by her parents.

What were less understandable, though, were Alison's references to other aspects of her parents whom she continually tried to ennoble. She spoke of her mother as a 'wonderful mother', 'who would do anything for her family'. Her father was 'really soft' about his daughters. A few minutes later she would be describing her father putting his hand in her knickers or her mother slapping her and laughing. The grandiose phrases used to describe the parents stood in marked contrast to the details of everyday cruelty and misery. Yet, Alison seemed unaware of these contradictions. It was possible for minutes at a time to have a conversation with her about her wonderful family and her bitterness at the social worker's interference. In this version of events 'social services' broke up their 'happy home' and myself and people like me had no idea what we had spoiled or what rubbish we offered instead. As long as I listened to this and refused to play the role of 'interfering authority' she would end the diatribe against 'do-gooders' by eventually running out of steam. Then, within minutes, she would sadly and plaintively refer to some aspect of her past life which filled me with horror. By the end of the session I was filled up with emotions which were hopelessly incompatible. How was I to draw to her attention the madness of these contradictory ideas, I wondered. Unbearable incompatible feelings of hatred and attachment, of abuse and dependence, of alienation and belonging were poured into me. 'You find a way out of this mess' seemed the unconscious request as she left, feeling 'better', whilst I was definitively 'worse'.

Alison could argue with her social worker that she wanted to return to her mother as 'no one understood how they loved each other'. Our understanding of attachment under duress is useful here. Insecure attachment is sometimes fiercer than ordinary good attachments. The debate about how memory works and whether patients like Alison can be described as having false memories is an important one. It has brought to attention the constructive aspects of memory (Sinason 1998).

The fact that memory is a reconstruction links it to the context in which one is having the memory and the possibility of different aspects being highlighted at different times. My experience as a therapist is that memories are not immutable. But neither are they infinitely malleable. What accounts for much of the debate about accuracy is that memories involve emotions both in the past and in the present. Under the sway of loss or loneliness we will recount an event differently than we do in anger or despair. I have not found, except with extreme episodes of mental disorder, that memories are false or totally absent and must be recovered. What I do find is that the emotional content and the meaning and significance of events can undergo change. What are repressed and liable to distortion are the feelings attached to an event. When these feelings are painful beyond bearing there seems to follow an inability to integrate emotions into an overall attitude. Alison could not present her relationship to her mother coherently. The failure, it seems to me, is not of memory *per se*; it is a failure of being able to rule definitively over opposing emotional needs. Thus Alison's attachment needs were heightened by her mother's absence and made her long for reconnection, made her ignore her abusive memories or seek to minimise their significance.

Self-abuse as a response to sexual abuse

Young people like Marilyn can harm themselves with drugs recklessly poured into themselves as if the risk of death were nothing. In this way they seem to be acting out an abusive relationship with themselves in both roles, abuser and victim.

Marilyn felt she needed another person who was more real and more worthy than herself to deflect the glances of others. If she was looked at she believed others would see her as peculiar and unlikeable. This made her an easy prey to men who treated her badly. In many ways she found such men a relief because they fitted in with her idea of herself and did not provoke self-examination or change in her. A split-off part of her identified with these bullies and gave her a sense of mastery over vicarious aggression which was her only satisfaction.

Another young woman, Paula, did not need a man to beat her up, she regularly cut herself when the feeling of 'not-rightness' became too much for her to bear. She described self-cutting as a deliberate violation of herself, cutting into her own body at the boundary of the skin. She believed she could let some of the bad feelings out with her blood, an action that held some appeal for early medicine, let us remember. But the meaning of this as symbolic sexual abuse with herself as perpetrator and victim also seemed likely from her descriptions. The angry, bloody display of herself to her foster carers also seemed to have a meaning of 'Look what has happened to me. Call yourselves parents?' It was perhaps a belated and misplaced indictment of the original parents' failure. The wounds inside that cannot be seen were exported out to horrify others. Paula did express some satisfaction, some revenge by this display. Yet other girls harm themselves in secret, hinting, almost teasing, therapists like me. The self-harm seems to continue their original abuse at the hands of someone more powerful. Now they are 'in control' and experience a masochistic satisfaction. Split off from their awareness, the sense of pain and concern which they have lost is felt by the therapist or foster parent. The frustration and powerlessness of others to intervene in this process can mean that the other is made to experience their own powerlessness from long ago.

Sexually abused children present a wide spectrum of personal and relationship difficulties that takes many months and years of careful understanding if they are to find their way back to non-abusive relationships and personal growth.

Chapter 7

The longing in belonging

Analytic neutrality

– attachment disorders
– adhesive relationships
– therapy in transition
– therapeutic breaks revive earlier losses
– adaptation of therapy rules in taking things out of sessions
– identification with the aggressor
– counter-transference of trauma
– pacing interpretation

Children who undergo the rupture of having to leave their birth family and live with foster carers or in a residential home suffer an enormous blow to their sense of belonging. They inevitably react as if they are to blame and emotionally they receive this event as a rejection, a punishment and a blow to their self-esteem. This was not at all clear to me when I first began working with children resident in a local authority community home in 1981. I thought then more about the escape these children had made from abuse, from harm, from danger. Naively I imagined that most children would feel rescued and look forward to a life free of abuse. As this was the exception rather than the rule it is still perhaps worth asking the question why. It does defeat logic to hear children yearn for a mother who neglected or beat them or to cling to a brutal abusive father.

The psychoanalytic approach emphasises that the first task is to listen and to be non-judgemental in terms of approval or blame, simply to let the feelings emerge and to try to understand. Of all the tenets of the psychoanalytic method this must be the most useful touchstone. We are not priests giving moral or ethical guidance. We are not teachers helping the child to learn by demonstrating useful truths. We are not counsellors giving helpful advice about what to do.

Analytic neutrality means that we have to 'get alongside' our patients, see things from their point of view, allow them to lead whilst we follow. We must be slow to judge or counsel or teach. Only then will less acceptable feelings emerge into the relationship.

Most of the children whom I met were very ambivalent about their 'removal to a place of safety'. Some regarded it as an unmitigated disaster and hated and blamed their social worker for taking them away. If one listened hard, though, most children held contradictory and incompatible beliefs about this event. They continued to hold contradictory and incompatible beliefs about returning home as well and this showed in their behaviour as well as their words. They could neither live with nor live without their families.

Matthew, 6 years

Six-year-old Matthew had no wish to go to an adoptive home and wanted to wait in the children's home until his mother one day returned. Mother was a teenage girl whose lifestyle revolved around drug addiction. She had eventually relinquished him and moved to another part of the country. Matthew fought off any attempts by adults to get close to him and severely tested the capacities of his adoptive parents. In therapy he busied himself with robots and tank warfare. Hard outer shells with many protective layers were the theme of his unwilling engagement with me. Only grudgingly did he let me participate in these games. My soldiers were trying to make peace and I put to him their dilemma, which was of course my own. They were knocking on the door of a tank trying to communicate but always being mistaken for enemies and attacked. Matthew hid his attachment to me so well that I only knew from others that he was angry on one occasion when illness prevented me seeing him. He told me he did not notice when we had interruptions to our twice-weekly sessions. Themes in his play always suggested, however, that he regarded absence on my part as trickery, as provocation to his jealousy, and he monitored with extreme vigilance any hints of my involvement with others in preference to him.

Donna, 10 years

By contrast, 10-year-old Donna seemed determined to like me immediately. She made a 'paper girl' in her early sessions which she kept in her therapy box and fed with paper food. Thin and desperately needy herself, Donna seemed to come close simply to feel my warmth. She often shivered with cold, seemed permanently under-dressed and malnourished. Never daring to complain, she seemed to accept whatever I gave without demur. Her wish to attach herself to me seemed to be symbolised by extensive endeavours to stand the paper girl up by trying to stick her to something stronger. The paper girl never seemed to be able to take much in as she was two-dimensional. Donna came and went easily from her sessions, friendly to everyone and no one in particular within the children's home. Eager, adaptable, a ready victim, her relationships were superficial and orientated to material things. She seemed to portray a form of 'adhesive' relationship to me (see Glossary).

It makes sense perhaps to think of Matthew and Donna as exhibiting two different insecure attachment styles (see Glossary). Matthew as 'insecure avoidant' shows the characteristic features of hiding his attachment, seeming aloof and unfeeling, giving little sign of how he reacts to my departure and reunion with him. I have watched videos of children like him at 1 year of age in the 'strange situation' task which Mary Ainsworth and others refined (Ainsworth and Wittig 1969; Ainsworth *et al.* 1978). This research put 1-year-old children into a situation where their mothers left them alone in a strange room for a few minutes. On the mother's return the child's behaviour was noted and categorised as evidence of an attachment style. On video it is now possible to gather a very detailed observation of the child's behaviour. What seems from a distance to be the child 'not noticing' the mother's departure and return is revealed in these videos as the child controlling their responses to mother's movements. Far from being unaware the child looks hypervigilant but lets out little expression or communication of this to mother. The child's preoccupation with mother's absence shows nonetheless in their inhibition of play or activity whilst she is gone. When she returns the child's eyes search her out but immediately look away, as if uninterested. Some moments later the child routinely makes a fuss about some seemingly incidental event, for example, that their shoe is undone, and they will often cry at that point. The mother, who is characteristically unaware of her child's feelings, interprets the child's initial responses as confirmation of her belief that 'he does not mind my absence' and often gets angry at what she perceives is inexplicable fussing over, for example, a shoe. Thus the scene is set for ongoing miscommunication and denial of loss (Parkes *et al.* 1991; Goldberg *et al.* 1995).

Donna is perhaps an example of 'insecure resistant' attachment. At one year in the 'strange situation' such children seem inconsolable at mother's return, often passively whining over long periods. It is as if their feelings over their abandonment are stretched out thinly and never quite brought to a head. Instead of protest followed by comfort (secure attachment) the child's protest seems muffled and ambiguous. Comfort is either not effectively offered by the caregiver or does not seem to be received by the child. An uneasy sense of muffled criticism seems to me to characterise the interaction.

Within child psychiatry 'attachment disorders' of childhood have been part of symptom classification since the 1990s and are included in the *International Classification of Diseases*, tenth edition (ICD10, World Health Organisation 1992). Two main kinds of attachment disorder are postulated: one 'ambivalent attachment' and the other 'indiscriminate attachment'. Matthew and Donna in my example would be considered to fit these two categories of attachment disorder respectively.

The simplicity of attachment categories is both appealing and frustrating. They do serve to alert us to an important dimension in the past experiences of fostered children and their stance toward parents old and new. These children's security in relationships is a key dimension and often a key deficit in the way that they relate throughout their lives. Attachment research also convincingly predicts infant attachment styles from mother's responses to the Adult Attachment Interview. In this latter interview, the mother's ability to give an emotionally integrated and coherent account of her own childhood predicts security in her infant's attachment one year later with 70–80 per cent accuracy (van Ijzendoorn 1995; Main 1991: 127). The child's internal version of their relationships is, however, a more varied and complex story. This can be illustrated by the case of Polly, a little girl in a three-year, once-per-week therapy.

Polly, an abandoned child

Polly was a thin, nervous, 8-year-old when I met her for the first time. She hesitated before she accepted my invitation to sit together at the table and draw a picture. She wanted me to draw too. She seemed prim and careful, using a ruler to mark out the outline of an insubstantial house.

Polly's pictures contained fragments of four different homes which she told me about. This was how she started our once-weekly therapy. Polly had been in several different foster homes whilst her young mother intermittently managed to care for her. In one of the many placements in her past she had been sexually abused by a knife-wielding teenager. In a later placement she had been found sexually abusing a smaller child and she was swiftly removed to another placement.

When I first met her, Polly was in a 'bridging placement' that was meant to prepare her for adoption. In a recurrent dream she told me about much later, she was always lost, running everywhere, trying to find someone to whom she belonged.

The literature about 'attachment' points to an abiding human need for young, developmentally immature children to have emotional safety with parents. In Polly and children like her we find that 'attachment' is putting the need mildly. Belonging is what human children crave. Without belonging we hardly know who we are, we scarcely know where to begin. Here is how Polly expressed it in the early stages of therapy.

> 'You can play with this family and they live in the doll's house,' she says as she allocates the family dolls to me. She takes for herself several big animals and dinosaurs. They watch from a distance as she tells me to make the family sit down at a table to eat. The big animals hesitatingly approach. 'We're so hungry. We haven't eaten for days. We've got no home,' she makes them say. They 'camp' near the family and the family feed them. Polly says, 'The animals aren't mean, they're just very hungry . . . and big.' At night she tells me to put the family to bed and to sleep. Other creatures join the nearby camp and want food as well. They all go into the kitchen and raid it and make a mess. The 'dinosaur bird' is Polly's favourite. 'It's silly that people are afraid of spiders because they are bigger than them and probably the spider is more scared than the people,' she tells me, although there is no spider in her play. The family continue to have trouble with the 'camp', sometimes being bitten, always being raided for extra food. 'They're just big and they've got no food or home,' Polly reiterates. She is very matter of fact. Toward the end of the session I tell her we will have to end in five minutes. 'All the creatures have to go back to where they come from,' she says. They howl and hop and flap and grumble and snarl away. 'Huh, it wasn't such a good camp,' she makes one say. I try gently to comment that Polly finds it very disappointing to stop and that she feels rejected and pushed away by me. She will have none of it and says on the contrary that 'it seemed too long today'.

I thought that Polly used big, ugly, fierce creatures to represent herself and her need for shelter. There was acknowledgement of the difficulty and mess that such overwhelming need creates in 'the family'. But she claimed the motives of the needy creatures were simply for food and shelter: their anger was simply in response to rejection. Polly seemed to be puzzling about being perceived as frightening even though she herself is small like the spider. Her sense of her own ugliness is profound. She seemed, also, desperate for someone to overcome this perception of her and to see the hungry child within.

We can see how painful it is for the session to stop in the midst of these feelings. There is an immediate assumption of rejection as the animals howl and retreat. The acerbic comment that it was not such a good camp betrayed Polly's defence against what she felt was my rejection. She criticised what was on offer and denied that she really wanted it. By claiming the session was too long she attempted to invoke in me feelings of being unwanted and rejected.

If the story were this simple, foster and adoptive parents would have little difficulty taking in a child like Polly. Her need for a home would soon find welcoming parents. But underneath the neediness and fear of rejection there are often other more malignant feelings. In Polly's case she was desperate to be seen as 'ordinary' in her life at school and in the foster home. Inside she hid her deep mistrust of adults, her anger and rebellion at her fate, her wish to be exceptional. Perceiving that many of her feelings were nasty and unacceptable she was at pains to hide them well and to deny them to herself. The problem with such a strategy is that she became out of touch with these difficult feelings which were nevertheless picked up by others as falseness, as slyness, as superciliousness. It is hard genuinely to like a child who is afraid of being genuine. The therapeutic hour is an opportunity to have revealed some of this inner turmoil with limited repercussions, to take the chance of being really known.

Each therapy session has a beginning, a new chance perhaps to start again. A child psychotherapist allows the patient to begin each meeting. Of course, there may be continuity of themes or the child may start where they left off, but the therapist ensures that she does not impose a continuity that cancels the chance of starting somewhere else or leaving alone the conversation of the last meeting. This is left to the patient to determine. Each therapy session has also an end, a goodbye, a break. The experience of endings and breaks is often particularly painful for these patients whose lives are full of catastrophic endings. Despite my enhanced sensitivity to these feelings from working with this group of young people I was still shocked when, coming up to our first Christmas break, Polly suddenly asked me at the end of the session: 'Will I be coming back here after Christmas?' At that time I had known her for nine months and had carefully explained the length of each break we had. It is at these moments that I realise again how fragile is these children's sense of security and how at each turn they expect me simply to disappear. I would be horrified to act in such a cavalier fashion whilst they seem to expect it. Polly not only expected me to drop her but she compliantly played to the end of her session despite believing that I would do so.

Many children with broken attachments insist on taking things in and out of the therapy sessions. The usual rule in analytic psychotherapy is that the pictures and products of each session remain in the child's box in the therapy room. This is to underline the symbol of containment that the therapist will take care of what emerges in the room and will look after things until the next meeting. It also acts as a message of confidentiality, that the products of the session are private between therapist and patient. However, children with histories like Polly's have a different agenda and one that may need to be acknowledged and allowed by the therapist. They find it hard to believe that they will return, that their things will be looked after, that they can trust the therapist to come back. The session endings may feel for a long time as if they are a confirmation of their experience of rejection. The little items that many such children bring to and fro may be the child's attempt to establish continuity and to bridge one session to another. Therefore Polly, when told that she could not take away her session drawings began to bring in a series of her own playthings. They were mainly a number of tiny 'creatures': a 'mouse' she had fashioned out of a piece of stone, a hairslide with a bunny on it, a 'troll' she had bought with her pocket money. These little figures took up residence in her box for a short while and then went back into her pocket and to her foster home. From time to time she swapped them over. Thus the wish to stay with me was acted out and interwoven with an experience of coming and going. She left with me something to link herself back to me. She took away tiny creatures that had been in my care. Transitions were difficult for Polly and she worked hard at holding herself together during them. In her art work and in her stories she sought integration and continuity. Her keen sense of history was shown from her first drawing and later in the integrity of her play characters' personalities. Perhaps this is why in her therapy she favoured the dinosaur bird, a creature from the past. It was a toy with moveable wings, a sharp beak and huge talons.

By the eleventh month of her therapy Polly had filled out many details of her games with this dinosaur bird. This is an extract from my notes toward the end of our first year:

> She wanted the doll's house on the table between us and soon set up a story. I was asked to take the part of the little dolls, whom she instructed me, were 'an ordinary family'. Polly was to be three animal babies, the baby kangaroo, the monkey and the dinosaur bird. I described all of these to Polly in terms of her former games with them, checking with her to see if I had understood correctly. The monkey was cheeky and lived without a family but got along on his wits. She made him a clever teasing animal who went easily from

> one group to another. The baby kangaroo no longer lived in her mother's pouch but was tiny enough to trick larger creatures and escape triumphantly. The dinosaur bird, I said carefully, was seen by others as ugly – 'It is ugly,' she quickly corrected me. The story began with a human family moving into a new home. They do not realise that three creatures are already living in the attic. Polly carefully pushed her toys in the doll's house attic, out of sight. The monkey is the first to be discovered. The family are charmed by him and Polly suggests that they will let him live with them. He makes mischief and a lot of mess but the family find him so comical they easily forgive him. 'Monkeys are cute,' Polly says to me. The monkey's friends show themselves only to the human children and ask them not to tell their parents but to let them live secretly with the family. Life goes on with lots of adventures for the children, including exciting and dangerous rides on the back of the dinosaur bird. The mother and father are unaware of all this activity. I discuss with Polly the meaning of the bird who seems to represent a part of herself that cannot fit in, that is mistrustful of adults and wants to do exciting, perhaps dangerous, things. She immediately reacts to the implication of this and denies that she did anything sexual to her sister at her adoptive home, 'It was a mistake and they just thought she did.' She hurries on with the game. The bird gets fed up of not being as liked as the kangaroo and monkey and one night brings 'his mates' to the house. They are a whale and an alligator. These animals bite up the children and the parents and the story disintegrates into chasing, eating, resaving, recapture whilst the home is destroyed. 'Who are these others, where do they come from – the whale and the alligator?' I ask. 'Oh you remember,' she replies, 'they used to be in a gang with the dinosaur.' In the middle of the devastation she suddenly says, 'The dinosaur doesn't want to be in with the gang any more. It wants to be in a family and learn how to behave.' She cuts across anything I may say by hurriedly clearing the toys away and announcing she is going to play 'something different'.

We can see in this play a more complex scenario than a needy child who wants to belong to a family. I perceived the three attic dwellers as representing different aspects of Polly herself. Perhaps they are in the attic of the house because in the top of herself, in her head and mind, she is aware of hidden allegiances. There is a strong and repeated theme in her play of one acceptable aspect being 'on show' whilst two further aspects are hidden and disruptive. Thus the adults in the household meet the monkey but are unaware of his link to the less acceptable kangaroo and the ugly and exciting dinosaur bird. The children meet the dinosaur bird but are unaware of his link to a yet more destructive whale and alligator. The monkey can be thought of as a survivor, clever, perhaps manipulative, getting into mischief but always charming and forgivable. This may have been Polly as she would like to be seen. The baby kangaroo is a more fragile, motherless child. Tiny and really belonging with a mother, his fragility is denied by Polly whilst he seems omnipotently to triumph over his adversaries. In some games he would be in the midst of a battlefield and able to get onto a bigger creature's back and bite them and still escape through a tiny exit. The dinosaur bird was Polly's unacceptable side. This is a creature who is ugly. It is a creature with a history. The bird's wish to belong is ambivalent because he does not trust the grown-ups of the family. He has habits of an exciting dangerous nature that the adults do not know about but that the children join in. Perhaps spurred on by my discussion of this dinosaur bird Polly reveals that his allegiances are still to aggressive wild creatures – 'the gang'. A gang it seems is an alternative to a family: it is a delinquent non-parented group who keep together against the adult world. The gang rob from and attack the family using their deprivation to justify their lawlessness. Polly's dinosaur bird is in a quandary, it seems. The bird is shunned by parents, seen as ugly, fearful of constant rejection. It falls back on old malign allegiances. But in this session in the middle of the gang's destructive attack on the family Polly says, 'The dinosaur doesn't want to be in with the gang any more. It wants to be in a family and learn how to behave.'

Polly's wish for parents and mistrust of parents was a constant theme in her play. Her relationship to me was therefore something she struggled with, as she felt she must constantly defend herself against me. Trying to help her acknowledge some of her anger and despair I was constantly warned by her that she was not sure she wanted to keep coming to therapy. She watched me keenly in my response to the delinquency of some of her play, and was clearly relieved at my refusal to condemn aggression but to seek to understand it. When I occasionally laughed at some 'naughtiness' of a character she warmed to me and made up games where we were 'twins' who set up home in 'the wilderness'. These child-only worlds quickly became self-help organisations. The children tucked each other into bed at night, shared the cooking and housework, settled each other's fears and comforted each other. They were not a gang and hardly a delinquent sub-culture. They just did without adults. But she was always the controlling character in these games, the one who knew what to do. I was allocated a role of follower, of dependant. Trust and intimacy were therefore things that Polly could only have if she were in control. She could not trust an equal or a more powerful adult.

These themes of our being twins seemed relatively benign attempts at friendship in a child struggling to adapt to her motherless state. Who, with her experiences, would not wish for a relationship where the trauma of rejection and abuse would be minimised and controlled? In her life outside the therapy room she began to cry for the adoptive mother and father who had abandoned her. She reiterated at her review meetings her conscious wish for a family to whom she could belong.

Trauma and its aftermath

In her defensiveness, her wish for control, her need for and fear of attachment, Polly was like many children whose histories have left them ambivalent and mistrustful of adults. There was a different and altogether more sinister quality, however, to certain aspects of her therapy. Tiny glimpses of cruelty appeared and were quickly covered over in her play. She simply looked blank at my tentative attempts to point these out. Then, following the material of the three creatures in the attic, Polly cleared away this game and swiftly set up another.

There were three boats full of swimmers and I was told they were out in the sea at night. Because it was dark they could not see what was in the water and did not realise they were completely surrounded by a gang of fierce predators (this was Polly's own description to me including her word 'predators'). The predators were all different so the people in the boats were giving each other warnings that only served to confuse. 'There's a walrus with great big tusks coming towards you on your right!' one boat would shout to another. But it was not a walrus, it was a whale that was attacking the boat and not from the right but from the left. The boat therefore moved into the path of its predator. People got out of the boat to swim in the sea. Swimmers were therefore killed and eaten in the dark. The predators were of every shape and size. The people were endlessly pursued and eaten up. People in the boats kept mistaking their enemies or, even when they saw them, thought them less aggressive or dangerous than they turned out to be. For example, they saw the fin of the big shark, one of the fiercest predators in Polly's game, and they thought it was the fin of a dolphin. They got happily into the water to play with the dolphin and were torn limb from limb as they were eaten in silence. The feeling was one of nightmare. Polly dispatched each person with quiet, chilling care. Silence underlined each death. The game was hurriedly put away without words but with so much banging of the toys and cupboard doors that my words were drowned out as she insisted on leaving early.

When she had left I felt quite shaken. I was left in no doubt that something awful, something chilling and inhuman, had been shown to me. The impact of this material lodged itself in me to the degree that I felt I had shared part of the experience. The coldness, the silence of the scene, where in the dark, unspeakable nightmare grips the swimmers. Something in the grave way she dispatched the people, the absence of grief, of pity, caused me to shudder. The attempts of the people to defend themselves seemed pathetic and were doomed to failure. Their naivety, their reasoning, was altogether inadequate for their situation. They were attacked by cold-blooded murderers. After the story Polly rushed out, seeming afraid of me.

I went back after this session to Polly's file and found myself re-reading her interview by a child psychiatrist following her disclosure of sexual abuse. I read of Polly who at the age of 4 years had a teenage boy climb into bed with her and threaten her with a knife. He told her that he would kill her if she did not keep silent whilst he sexually assaulted her. She had kept silent. She had endured in terror. Had some kind of fragmentation of herself occurred so that she felt surrounded by many enemies? Was this teenage boy the only predator in that chaotic household or was she surrounded by others who would abuse her in the dark?

In Polly's therapy session the innocent playful swimmers meet their death under the surface of normality in the silence and dark of night. The stuff of nightmare was haunting 9-year-old Polly in a foster home, whilst she consciously wanted a family to whom to belong.

The context in which this traumatic predator story comes up in Polly's session is important. It follows the part of the session when the 'dinosaur bird' has evoked his past allegiance to 'the gang' and this has destroyed the happy family. Polly has commented that 'it wants to be in a family and learn how to behave'. She puts away those toys and takes out the boats and swimmers. Nightmare follows. Haunted by an experience she cannot process and that she fears to talk about, Polly is showing me the obstacle to her belonging to a new family.

I was left in no doubt through my own feelings in the counter-transference how difficult and painful Polly found it for me to address this material. There must have been apprehension on her part that I was a friendly dolphin-like person who could turn out to be another attacker, perhaps the worst of all. She must have feared my insight and my ability to see her in the dark. I felt that, above all, I had to be very gentle in order not to add to her fright. I let her leave that session early, as she insisted.

I wanted her to know that I would not force her to do anything. I let her silence me then and often did so when she could not bear me to comment. I did not set the agenda, I followed hers so that she could control a process I know caused her pain.

In her therapy session the next week Polly wanted me to be a doctor to whom she was bringing a child to have an injection. She, as the 'child's mother', explained that she knew it would hurt but the child needed it in order to get better. She asked me, 'Shall we say it doesn't hurt although it does a bit?' She watched me very closely as I replied that we should tell the child the truth, even if it was a difficult truth. I could see her visibly relax as I admitted the pain of my healing treatment.

Having gone so far and evidently feeling too exposed, Polly backed away from these difficult themes for a while. Or perhaps it happened that these more violent thoughts abated. She immersed herself in stories about animal families where babies are abandoned, but eventually, after many vicissitudes, reunited with loving relatives. She played out many variations of how mother and father and baby become separated. Sometimes the mother goes off on an adventure. Sometimes she is ill and dying. Sometimes she intends to return but gets delayed. There was an innocent kindly feeling to these stories which came out all right at the end. The tenacity of the animals in always striving toward their home and their kin was remarkable. Like the adventures of Ulysses, these stories had an epic, timeless quality.

But, of course, they had a personal, poignant meaning given Polly's 'refugee' status. This is one example from when Polly had been in therapy for a year:

> Two horses have a baby together. The nursing mother is put into a different field from the father. He goes off. One morning the mother is gone. The baby does not know why. She is looked after by other animals. Time passes and baby is as big as her mother. Then one day two visiting horses gallop past. One visitor looks just like this one. The other animals think they must be ghosts. But gradually they get to know these 'new horses'. It turns out they are the mother and father horse returned.

In following sessions Polly began again a series of stories that developed over many sessions and which followed the theme of predatory danger. Here is an excerpt from her second year of therapy:

> Polly took a large crocodile out and said he was in a field but hidden from view. Into the field was thrown an assortment of animals, all

> small, mainly baby lambs and calves. Polly tells me that they have just been put in there to feed the crocodile but they don't realise it. They don't know he lives in the field. One of the 'babies' is a young zebra and Polly tells me, 'You can be the mother zebra because people can see that it misses its mother,' and she adds a large zebra to the field. She asks me whether I have hairs on my legs: 'Grown-up ladies can do, can't they and it means that they're strong?' A friend of the foster carer had told her this, she said.

In the game the little animals venture out into the field to play. Wide-eyed and innocent, the first ones to venture near the crocodile get eaten up. The zebra baby tells its mother who then realises what is going on and makes a shelter for all of the animals. 'She looks after all the babies, not just the zebra', Polly explains. The crocodile goes blind and can only smell and hear the animals. Mother zebra warns them to stand stock-still if he touches them: one baby manages this but another screams in fright. She is eaten. The mother zebra scolds: 'I told her to keep quiet.' One baby lamb is quiet but still is smelt and eaten. I keep up a commentary on the horribleness of these events. I describe aloud the babies' innocence and fear. How awful it must be to live with an enemy so close by. Polly tells me that the zebra's hard hooves can hurt the crocodile and the mother zebra also wrests some of the babies from the crocodile's mouth. At the end of the session Polly is reluctant to leave and gives to me a little cat she has made from a piece of cloth. She says to me, 'Do you think you could have this to look after?'

There followed a steady stream of games where animals lived in a 'field' or in the sandpit and 'predators' were nearby. The predators began steadily to lose the battle. The strong mother zebra was sometimes joined by other 'mothers' who united to protect the young. Separations of mothers and babies frequently occurred, with attendant danger to the babies. In the sandpit young animals were put there 'to fatten them up for the predators'. The main predator was the dinosaur bird who flew overhead inspecting his prey.

Three months later and the story continued:

> 'We'll put the animals in the desert again to be fattened up for the predators,' Polly announces. The mother zebra and mother giraffe successfully protect them when the dinosaur bird swoops down, trying to carry off the young. 'They're going to take the mothers out now because the predators are going hungry and don't like it.' I ask who makes these decisions and who are 'they'? 'No one knows,' she

> tells me evenly. The young now have to defend themselves. They help each other to remember how the mothers built strong defences in the sand. Together they outwit the predator bird. I talk about the situation of Polly at the abuser's home and how much she needed a mother to protect her. 'Yes, but I've forgotten all about that now. I never think of that now,' she replies. She does not seem to mind my wondering aloud whether it felt like this. She looks thoughtful and her game ends with the predators 'going away to pick on someone else'.

Gradually then I could talk with Polly about her hope for a protective parent who would not deny the danger or pain but help her to protect herself. As Polly began to believe in a maternal force in me that sought to protect her so she became hopeful of learning self-protection. I was careful in this role not simply to act in the way that Polly dictated. The incident of the mother zebra criticising the terrified child for 'making a noise' I challenged. I carefully 'thought out loud' that it could not be the youngster's fault for being attacked. However young and silly someone is, it does not excuse predatory attack. I said that aggression is always the problem of the perpetrator who must learn to take responsibility for controlling it. In these discussions I sought to correct Polly's false attributions of blame. She was not to blame for her own abuse but neither, in the foster home, was her little victim to blame.

In this way I came again to focus on the part played in Polly's stories by the dinosaur bird. This creature early on in our sessions was an ugly rejected creature who had been a gang member. We know that Polly closely identified with this bird which mainly seemed to represent a part of herself she felt other people were afraid of and rejected. In her early play the bird involved itself in exciting dangerous games with other children. These activities were unknown to the parents. The bird was also attached to destructive angry forces, a whale and a crocodile. Was this the part of Polly which pursued and sexually abused a child of whom she was jealous? In her foster home she had forced small toys inside this little girl's vagina, threatening her to silence, pretending she had a knife as her own abuser had. It was the discovery of this behaviour which struck abhorrence into foster parents and led them to have her removed. How could she own this part of herself which had driven away parents that she was desperate to retain? But the dinosaur and its history continued to follow her. It was both a persecutor like the boy who sexually abused her and an identification which led her to abuse another child.

In the play of the predator in the desert the dinosaur bird reappears as a creature who seeks to hurt and devour the vulnerable. If it is unclear with which creatures Polly identifies in this play, this may be because she is predator as well as prey. If I as therapist precipitately condemned violence this would have left Polly stranded with a violent part of herself she was at pains to disown. Colluding with her violence would be equally problematic, for it would be to deny the aggressor's power and to condone her own abuse of long ago. I therefore took very seriously the problem of my attitude toward the dinosaur bird and let Polly know that I remembered all the parts of his history. She agreed that he was the same bird who 'had once lived in the family's attic'. Gradually we denied this bird the right to have the motherless young. The babies took on an identification with a strong father-like mother (with hairy legs!). Fathers started to appear in the play to strengthen the mother's position and help protect the young. Polly began to explore different sorts of families in her play, being very fond of elephants 'who mate for life and the dads don't go off and leave the mums'. We were sometimes, but only when she was willing, able to discuss her ideas about her own young mother whose abandonment led to her unprotected life in an abusive family. The dinosaur bird 'got fed up of never having any meat and became a vegetarian'. Gradually she excluded it altogether from her play.

It took three years for Polly to be able to talk about her history in a realistic way. Her fears and her trauma continued to inhibit some aspects of herself and her memories always had to be approached with caution. She was still quick to deny links to her past. But gradually she was able to own her own aggression and to work to contain it rather than simply hide it.

In this way Polly came to identify with a strong protective parent in order to contain internal aggression and external threat. It is this identification, the taking inside of a protective parent, which gives the child a psychological home, a place where she belongs. Adoptive parents who wish to take in a child in this situation must also, it seems, accommodate the monster who hovers around the child. This monster part of the child is wary, aggressive, may be identified with an abuser or a bully, may belong secretly to a delinquent gang who have dispensed with the need for parents. It is this aspect of the child that causes most trouble and which the naive parent may not understand. There is no way to take in the sweet Polly who longs for a home without contending with the ugly restless predator with a poisonous bite.

Chapter 8

Identity in crisis

Damaged attachments

- negative identifications with parents
- abusive attachment
- internalised guilt
- the omnipotent defence
- persecutory anxiety
- repetition compulsion
- splitting
- reverence for the perpetrator
- long-term treatment needs
- resilience
- mental illness in a parent

'I love Auntie Precious for fostering me, but, oh, I hate being fostered,' 12-year-old Wayne said to me one day. 'If your mum don't deserve no respect then you don't either. . . .' Children identify with their parents and take their parents' attributions personally. My colleague child psychiatrist, Dr Anula Nikapota, told me of an incident where she was talking with school children about how to deal with name-calling. A little girl put up her hand with a question: 'You know when they say you're mum's a rude word and that? Well, what do you do if it's true?'

This is the dilemma felt by many looked-after children. Still, most children will defend their parents' name and thereby their attachment to them. It is often in adolescence that the looked-after children reveal how impelled they feel to renew their links with birth parents no matter how abusive or destructive such relationships may be. Foster parents and care professionals are on the receiving end of angry tirades that claim their care and protectiveness is abuse and 'spoiling their fun'. Carers have to stand on the sidelines whilst many of these young people run off, pour drugs and drink into themselves, expose themselves to rough sleeping, casual sex, abusive relationships with exploitative others, self-harm. Adolescents often frequent the neighbourhoods from which they originated, turn up on mother's doorstep, try to go home. These young people are rarely running away – they are running back (Wade *et al.* 1998: 65–8) If we set this behaviour in the context of attachment theory it begins to make more sense. The situation of a child with an attachment to an abusive parent is necessarily difficult to resolve as Main and Weston pointed out:

> The situation is irresolvable because rejection by an established attachment figure activates simultaneous and contradictory impulses both to withdraw and to approach. The infant cannot approach because of the parents' rejection and cannot withdraw because if its own attachment. The situation is self-perpetuating because rebuff heightens alarm and hence heightens attachment leading to increased rebuff, increased alarm and increased heightening of attachment.
>
> (Main and Weston 1982, quoted by Hopkins 1990)

Hopkins succinctly points out that 'the clinical outcome is an intense anxious dependency which is much harder to outgrow than the dependency experienced in a secure relationship' (Hopkins 1990: 460).

In other words, many of the children we see in foster or residential care have high dependency needs expressed in a pattern of insecure attachment. Just like the video of a poorly attached mother and child described in the last chapter, there is an ironic danger that such 'avoidant attachment' behaviour by a young person is perceived as 'independence'. Indeed, teenagers often characterise this behaviour to themselves as their wish to be free of parental influence from foster carers or social workers. If they are given such 'freedom' they routinely demonstrate their incapacity to keep themselves from harm. They run to meet danger, the professionals look on helplessly, thwarted in their attempts to parent. In this way, many abused children rescued from external danger in childhood go back to re-experience it during adolescence. Perhaps they are sometimes in touch with the repetition compulsion which seems to shriek 'Can't anyone stop this?' Similarly, sexually abused girls involve themselves with the first man they can find who will sexually exploit them. Their poor internal models of how relationships are conducted and their 'unconscious sense of guilt' (Freud 1973: 141) almost ensures the relationship's abusive nature, their failure and their repeated misery. These young people are often unconsciously (see Glossary) seeking punishment and abuse to fulfil an internal idea that they deserve misery. Poorly attached and badly treated children believe very strongly that this is their own fault, blaming themselves for their parents' failure to love them. Such children tend not to think 'my parents are deficient and cannot care for me'. They tend to think 'I am deficient and cannot be worthy of care'. The rage and aggression felt by a neglected or abused child cannot be channelled back toward the parent without fear of total abandonment. The child therefore often redirects this anger towards him- or herself, keeps the aggression within. Such an internal situation seeks punishment, blame, self-harm.

We can see from the example of Polly in the previous chapter that the sense of identity a child has can be troubled and complex. The child of adversity, of trauma, of broken attachments will find it hard to integrate the many aspects of his or her developing self.

There may be split-off pieces of the self which remain hidden, unacknowledged and out of the control of the young person. In 5-year-old patient Kirk's therapy (Hunter 1993b), I thought this was neatly symbolised in the following session:

> He arranged a 'lovely café' where two families came to have dinner. One was his adoptive family, the other 'Mrs Hunter's family'. When he had arranged a careful series of dolls around the table he pushed one boy doll aside. 'There isn't enough room,' he said, and pushed this boy into 'the dustbin'. During the meal, which he played out as a happy event with generous portions of food for all, the 'dustbin boy' got out and made attacks on the gathering, stealing food, throwing stones and pushing over their chairs.
>
> In earlier sessions he had played that a boy had been rescued from the burning building of his family by getting into a dustbin which was thrown out of the window to safety.

Kirk had in reality been accommodated when a fire in his house had rendered the family homeless. At 3 years of age his mother had blamed the fire on him and refused to have him any longer. The dustbin, I believe, was symbolic. It represented the fact that his mother had thrown him away, discarded and unwanted. Nevertheless this ejection from his birth family meant that he was 'saved', welcomed into a warm, accommodating adoptive family whose 'big portions' of food were well appreciated by Kirk. In his play his adoptive family and my family represent the generous, sharing, appreciative parts of Kirk. An earlier, angry part of himself is thought of as still living in the dustbin. This part believes there is no room for him at the happy gathering. Instead it attacks and tries to destroy the family's happiness.

Why is there 'no room at the table' for the rejected boy? In Kirk's case his therapy made clear it was because the dustbin boy continued to pursue a destructive vendetta against parents. The dustbin had been idealised into a strong, omnipotent protective shell which Kirk was loath to leave. He seemed less to believe (like Polly) that there were unacceptable parts of him that would lead to rejection than to be addicted to a triumphant 'I don't need anyone'. He played for many months with a character he called 'the stunt boy' who could perform wonderful tricks and 'stunts' on his bicycle. The stunt boy never got hurt – he always landed on his wheels. We can speculate that Kirk's original attachment to his mother must have been characterised by mistrust and fear of dependence. He had adopted a hard, angry, aggressive omnipotence to which he clung. It could be true that there is 'no room' at the family table for such an attitude.

Similarly with Polly: the delinquent gang of destructive animals with which she had felt comforted and identified had to be given up if she was 'to live with a human family'. There are losses, therefore, as well as gains in attachment to others and integration of the self. The potency of aggression must be relinquished. The fantasy of independence has to be humbled.

Much of therapy is concerned with observing and appreciating 'defence mechanisms' (see Glossary) which are used to protect the self from anxiety. Because many looked-after children are exposed to intense levels of insupportable fear their defences tend to be strong, rigid attitudes that repel many advances. The greater the danger, the stronger the fear, the weaker the child, the more do psychological means of protection have to create an illusion of bearable safety. Impotent fear is turned to illusory power, omnipotence. Dennis, who had been serially rejected by his mother, his father and his grandparents, having lived with each in turn, told me 'everyone in my family wants me to live with them. But I'm just going to stay in here [the children's home] for a while because I just can't choose who to live with!' This was delivered with a big empty smile. Nevertheless one felt Dennis would gradually be able to confide his fear that no one wanted him, so near did it seem to the surface. Zara, who grumbled about every assessment session 'because there is nothing wrong with me' rigidly denied that any fight or trouble she was in could be her responsibility. She felt the bruises she had inflicted on her adoptive mother's arms showed 'she just bruises easily' or 'she should not wind me up'. Zara at 12 years of age disowned her own hostility. She believed she lived in a hostile, complaining environment. She very effectively lodged her own sense of persecution into other people, especially her adoptive mother. It is uncertain with a young person like Zara, whose defences seemed watertight, whether these can be breached or loosened except in times of crisis. When the defences cause problems or get in the way of Zara's plans she may become motivated to consider therapy. Sadly, my assessment of her revealed that she felt I simply persecuted her and she adamantly refused my offer of further help.

Persecutory anxiety can be very difficult to relieve because clients like Zara feel threatened by any attempt to get close to them. Keeping a careful distance may lead to 'boredom' and denigration of the therapist for being 'useless'. These criticisms increase the inner fear of the young person that they will be, or should be, punished for their aggression and denigration. They try consciously or unconsciously to provoke punishment and rejection.

Naomi: living in two worlds

Naomi who was 15 came from a large, troublesome extended family who were well known to the police and the local inner-city social services department. Her grandparents, her grandmother's sisters, their four daughters and two sons, their various partners and their children lived in and out of each other's houses. Naomi lived with her single mother and mother's new husband who eventually regularly sexually abused Naomi. The extended family were constantly at war with each other. Factions of various members would gang up against others over a dispute. Then these alliances would founder over a further dispute and new allegiances and enemies were made.

When Naomi talked about her family she portrayed a preoccupation with trickery, disputes and alliances, violence and vendettas. A major theme of her accounts concerned who knew what, who told secrets to whom, who was loyal or disloyal. 'Secrecy' was endemic. Betrayal was frequent and inevitably led to a fight. Fights were exciting, dangerous affairs where one family member confronted another for their duplicity or mendacity. It was difficult in Naomi's excited and engaging renditions of these family dramas not to sit back wide-mouthed and entranced. She was a beautiful, vivacious girl of mixed-race appearance, jet-black long hair and golden-brown skin. Her father was unknown to her. Her white racist family alternately denied her mixed-race origins or rejected her for them. In this family attitudes to reality were as changeable as the alliances between members.

I began gradually to think of Naomi's accounts of this extended family as reflecting the state of Naomi's internal world, the state of her mind. Deep splits existed between the various parts of her. In one state of mind, for example, as a vitriolic bully, she was completely cut off from the pain of her victim. She was known for 'winding up' other girls, particularly a self-cutting girl who returned from escapades with Naomi in very bad states, often having lost a lot of blood. Yet Naomi herself was regularly beaten by her brutal boyfriends and continued to seek their acquaintance. This is an extract from one of our first sessions:

> She began by talking about an argument she was having with friends and how she would never let anyone do her down. A boy, Ryan, had put his hand up her skirt. She'd screamed and told him in no uncertain terms that she didn't let anyone do that to her . . . Her foster carers, Jo and Len, never seem to shout or grab, they are always so nice to each other . . . they do seem to have a good time though, like when they all went to holiday camp, a lot of fun. She didn't know that families could live together like that. But sometimes she feels she must run away for no reason, she can't even tell when she is going to do it or why . . . the other night she suddenly thought she'd go up to her home town, 40 miles away. She could easily hide in the toilet on the train and there was a train back at 11.30 p.m. Only, she missed it. She was a bit high, as they had cider earlier. She had phoned Jo, her foster mum, from the station. Instead of saying she was coming to get her, Jo had begun giving her a hard time about how worried they'd been when Naomi didn't come back home at 3.30 p.m. from school. Anyway Naomi had hung up. It was cool, she could stay with Claire and her man in a pretty good squat . . . Claire was 14 and her boyfriend about 30 but he was safe . . . The police raided for stolen goods. . . . And Claire and Naomi were arrested. It was Jo's fault, she should have come to pick her up, lazy cow, she's paid to look after her.

Some of this material was said quite provocatively and I certainly had the feeling that I was meant to disagree that staying in a squat with stolen goods, an abusive man and a young girl was 'safe'. There was, perhaps, an attempt to flaunt such risky and abusive scenarios in front of me. I think I was also perceived as like the middle-class foster parents who live in a 'nice' world where they act civilly to each other. Like them I am also paid to look after her. The gulf between the nice world and the 'squat' was very stark.

There would be several ways for the therapist to respond to this material. I could have drawn out the real relationships in Naomi's life and the contrasts and difficulties between them. Or I could concentrate on her relationship with me. Or a mixture of both to see what makes more sense to Naomi. What I would put in any account back to her is my understanding of the main themes of this material. I thought Naomi was telling me about a part of herself identified with her birth home and past which pulled her back to unprotected, risky but exciting, conditions. In that world there is no one to tell Naomi what she can and cannot do, and she can be high on drugs and drink, feeling powerful and free, which makes her miss her train, her link to a different life and different frame of mind. As in her past, there is a situation of an older exploitative male who has sex with a young girl. Naomi claims this situation is 'cool' and the man is 'safe'. This is the viewpoint of the past and of her family toward her abusive stepfather. Lack of protection, exploitation and neglect are denied as being painful. Naomi does attempt however to make a link from this state to her caring foster parents via the telephone. But the connection is tenuous. Naomi makes an outrageous claim on the foster carer who must drive an 80-mile round trip to pick her up, without being cross with Naomi. Naomi's anger and distrust of the carer emerges as it were in parentheses. If the foster mother cared she would come and get Naomi. Foster mother is accused of not caring, of being neglectful and lazy, of thinking only of money and not Naomi. Naomi therefore puts down the phone and cuts off from this attachment. At the same time Naomi pushes into the carer worries about her safety and Naomi's own anger and helplessness. One can imagine how foster mother felt at the other end of the phone.

In the relationship between Naomi and me, therefore, I could understand from this material that Naomi would try to make me bear the burden of concern, of rejection, of anger. She takes up a stance of mistrust of my motives, criticism of my laziness (sitting in my room whilst she is out in dangerous circumstances?), and despair that our connection will work. Yet, there is within this session a hope for a new attachment that can link Naomi's past and present, and that can rescue her from repetition of the past. There is a very little girl in Naomi who does have a hope that mummy will sort it all out. There is also a very little girl who is putting herself in danger as an attack on a mother she perceives as neglectful.

Psychoanalytic understanding of damaged attachments gives us a framework for grasping that it is not simply the offer of new, more secure, attachments that will help such young people. New attachments can all too easily be pushed into the same mould as old attachments. Naomi provoked anger, despondency and neglect in her carers. It was therefore critical to Naomi's future well-being that she grasped the repetition compulsion in herself. What was being repeated was a scenario where Naomi was in an unprotected situation with an abusive man whilst a mother 'looked on' from afar. Her perception of foster mother as uncaring, lazy and neglectful is a distortion of the present into the shape of the past. Her perception of herself as a helpless victim manipulated by more powerful others is similarly a distortion of reality. It is Naomi herself who has sought the danger she is in. Naomi was not conscious, however, of seeking out these repetitions, although she became wiser to herself over the course of her therapy. Naomi needed to understand her self-destructiveness as a complaint against a past mother. In identification with her abusive stepfather and her neglectful mother, Naomi was all set to make even very good carers powerless to help her.

One particular difficulty with Naomi's internal world was its changeablity. This was based on a very primitive way of functioning where good and bad events were simply experienced without being reflected upon, without being processed and integrated. Naomi's family seemed to embody the acting out of this kind of thoughtlessness. A friend today was an enemy tomorrow as soon as anything happened to disturb the relationship. With Naomi, I became aware that there was little attempt to integrate her opinions of people who were assigned characteristics according to their impact on her at that moment. Someone described to me as 'safe' and 'cool' on one day was suddenly referred to as 'that drug dealer who beat up Claire'. I do not mean that these descriptions changed as Naomi learned more about these characters. I mean that at any given time Naomi would seem to 'forget' things she knew about people. It was as if her emotional world were a kaleidoscope with few stable or secure features. Instead of working to integrate her opinions Naomi routinely did the opposite. She split her knowledge (see Glossary) into fragments. Much of the time she was quite out of touch with things that she knew in another frame of mind.

> Naomi began the twelfth session by telling me about a visit to her house from Claire's boyfriend, only Claire would not see him. Claire and she had told on him to the police but he didn't know. Claire was trying to dump him but he was really evil and bound to get nasty so she has to keep going out with him. She and Claire were going to get him locked up for a long time, they only have to say the word because he's dealing skag (heroin) and he can do a lot of time for that.

I establish that this is the 'safe' 30-year-old man that 14-year-old Claire was seeing some weeks ago. It is the same man that Naomi and Claire stayed with in the squat when Naomi ran away.

I remark that two things occur to me. One is that Naomi seems quite scared as she realises the kind of man she and Claire have become involved with. She tries to feel powerful when she thinks she can have him locked up but is meanwhile scared of his violence and is sensibly trying to keep away from him.

The second thing is that she had told me several times about this man without ever mentioning his violence and drug dealing. It's as if she keeps these pieces of information in different parts of her mind.

Naomi goes on to tell me about her stepfather visiting her sister. They seemed to get on OK. She wonders if she should let her social worker know that he's taking her younger sister out. She could stop it just by clicking her fingers but maybe her stepdad would get nasty to Naomi. I point out that the situation with Claire and with her sister are linked. Naomi's stepfather sexually abused Naomi over a long period. It seems that this knowledge is held separately from the knowledge that her younger sister will be alone with him. There is the same wish to be powerful by letting the authorities know and the same fear of retaliation by the abuser.

This leads to an extensive discussion about when Naomi lived with her stepfather and mother where it was known but not acknowledged by the family that he was raping Naomi. When Naomi finally told her social worker she was removed from her family, but family members continued to criticise her and call her a liar. She felt that she would lose contact with her family entirely unless she withdrew her allegations, so she had done so. She looked ashamed and admitted she couldn't stand up to them.

Perhaps from this session one can see Naomi struggling with a different kind of linking. Linking her thoughts, integrating her opinions against considerable external and internal forces against the process. It may have been impossibly painful for Naomi to have felt the full powerlessness of her life when she was at home. She buoyed herself up with an inflated idea of her power to have evil locked up. There was an important hope that, if someone knew, things would be different. One can sympathise that there was little external support to maintain this position. It seems ironic that Naomi feels ashamed and blames herself for not being able to take on her entire extended family. Sometimes, therefore, Naomi seems to have simply ignored what she knew, split it off into another set of feelings, as presumably did her family. This pattern of involvement with unsafe men was a strong habit of Naomi's that needed a great deal of work for her to recognise and perhaps finally to control.

Naomi was more victim than perpetrator in the examples above but there was a more destructive aspect to her when her identification with the abuser was uppermost. In a later session:

> Naomi spoke non-stop for the first ten minutes or so, excited and with much provocative 'Ooh, I must tell you! There was a fight – how it started was . . .'. Her mood was ebullient, even triumphant. She

> seemed to relish giving me details of her and her friend's involvement with sex, drugs and violence. I was aware of a fleeting feeling of being left out, dazed by a kind of anti-hero glamour in her talk. She was fully made-up, manicured and in tight black clothes, her long hair loose and constantly being flung back over her shoulder. She looked a picture of confident, youthful beauty. What she spoke of was a couple in her circle of friends who accused each other of being unfaithful. Two men had had a fight over this woman. Naomi thought this was hilarious, a real happening. Later the men made up and the woman got beaten for telling lies. Naomi is going out with the other man in the fight and doesn't believe he had sex with the woman. He is a traveller who no one would dare to mess about with, but he's 'sweet', he's just very jealous so she dare not look at anyone . . .

Gradually this session was brought to a more sober discussion of how violence and excitement can be used to make Naomi feel powerful. Allying herself to the violent jealous male allowed Naomi to feel she can 'ride the tiger' and not get hurt. She can enjoy the violence vicariously. I think in the transference relationship with me something else was being exchanged. Naomi was using me to play the part of a left-out person, envious, without sex, without excitement. Possibly I am meant to be the mother who has to relinquish sexual superiority to the daughter. The sexuality displayed is aggressive, jealous, violent, exciting. Naomi's pleasure in this sort of situation is real and makes her feel potent and triumphant. The real pain of a woman who gets beaten is denied. The brutality of the men is excused. It is not surprising to find in later sessions that Naomi is regularly beaten by this travelling man. She reveals this with shame but also believes that 'she deserves it'. There is a certain kind of emotional logic to her being 'punished' for her vicarious pleasure in other people's humiliation. It has little to do with reality, however, as this boyfriend will beat her regardless. Perhaps even her idea of deserving it is Naomi's last-ditch attempt to cling to an idea of her own powerfulness, her own belief in 'an eye for an eye'. In reality the violence Naomi receives is the undirected, casual aggression of a stronger, uncontrolled male over a girl who does not protect herself.

Naomi was an intelligent, challenging girl who came into therapy believing that she was fighting her way to freedom against the shackles of adult control. She became gradually aware that she was living a lie. The shackles were those of repetition compulsion. They were inside, not outside her. She found herself repeatedly in situations where she was being abused, in a drama where there were always three elements.

One was of a helpless, weak spectator. One was of a victim, often perceived as deserving punishment. The other was of a cruel and powerful male whose role must not be challenged. Naomi's attempts to 'tell' were attempts to activate the helpless mother who weakly looks on. It was a drama originating in real relationships within her family. But it became lodged inside her and in her identifications with each of the three personae: the victim, the manipulative bully, the watcher. As Naomi came to grasp a little more of her internal situation she became less defensively allied to the excitable high dramatics for which she was known. There were glimpses of the raw pain which she had fought to overcome:

> We had talked for much of the session about Naomi's worry that she was drinking too much and that she uses drink to be able to talk about her sexual abuse to her friends . . . after a sad silence she said suddenly, 'I've got this idea that I'd like to go back to my stepdad's room and steal something . . . I'd like to steal something he'd miss and keep looking for . . . I keep thinking of it.' I felt heavy with sudden sadness. He had taken from her this elusive thing. Something she missed and kept looking for that he had stolen, and that she could not find – her childhood, her trust, her innocence.
>
> Her loss welled up in me.

Kelly: 'My mother's a drunk, but a nice drunk'

Whilst Naomi had to find a voice, as it were, that was truly her own, her own identity outside of the repetitive abusive scenario of her childhood, another teenager, Kelly, seemed to have to choose between alternative identifications. Sixteen-year-old Kelly's mother was alcoholic. Her fondness for Kelly seemed genuine enough but it came second always to her fondness for alcohol. Kelly was a parentified child who seemed more mature, more forgiving and understanding than her mother. She called her mother 'a nice drunk'. In foster care Kelly began to thrive and to achieve academically in keeping with her intelligence. But her achievements were always haunted by the spectre of her mother. Kelly felt that at any moment she could 'become' her mother, drinking, crying, giving up hope. Kelly's struggle to achieve was made difficult by her fear of triumphing over her mother. Perhaps the child's long education in deflecting her own anger away from a mother who could not contend with it made Kelly unrealistic about her own power and her own culpability.

Hating her drunken mother she had tried to defend her, fearing to lose her entirely. She feared to criticise her or to be angry with her. In her unconscious mind Kelly hated her mother very much indeed and even feared that this was the cause of mother's weakness. It was not maturity but belief in her own culpability that governed Kelly's uncomplaining relationship to mother. The question became whether Kelly deserved to have a different life, a life of her own. Her fear was that this wish was an aggressive triumph over her mother. Could Kelly bear to be successful, to shake off her belief that she deserved to carry a burden?

Kelly was a quiet, self-effacing girl who did not complain. Her contrast with the loud-mouthed excitable Naomi could not be greater. But in her difficulty in believing in her self-worth and in her unconscious seeking of failure, they had much in common. Kelly was quietly carrying an identification with a sick mother where all aggressive elements of the relationship were strictly curbed and denied. In order to achieve for herself, this internal world had to be reorganised drastically. Kelly had to get gradually in touch with her anger and hatred of her mother. To some extent this was made possible by calling those elements of mother's behaviour which provoked rage and despair, 'mother's illness', or her 'drinking problem'. Kelly felt it was allowable for her to hate mother's drinking problem. She was deeply afraid of hating her mother. Kelly began gradually to see her difficulty with success as something that stemmed from an early wish to control and triumph over a despised mother. Her fear of success had to be disentangled from these early attempts to curb her own aggression.

Talking about feelings of anger, despair and hatred relieved Kelly very rapidly and helped her sustain academic pursuits. However, in the throes of exam anxiety, a different aspect of her identification with her mother emerged. Kelly revealed that she had a constant daydream that she could walk out of her exam room and all of what she called 'the pressure'. She could turn up at her mother's door and be taken in. They would have a few drinks together. At her mother's house, the dishevelled drunken environment had a comfort that was not present in the foster carer's neat and tidy home. Kelly would be able to flop down without questions, without expectations. Kelly's mother would not mind her daughter's lack of achievement, lack of striving for a future. Kelly imagined herself and her mother sharing the alcoholic haze and its comfort.

In this scenario Kelly used an identification with her mother to overcome anxiety about failure. Kelly felt the pressure of trying to achieve with its attendant pain of possible failure. No one, she felt, would criticise her for running to be with mother. Suddenly the much admired home of the foster carers felt alien to a girl filled with anxiety and fear that she cannot measure up. In this situation Kelly was revealing that her identification with her mother was not wholly self-sacrificial, not simply the wish not to harm her mother. It also functioned as a cloak for Kelly's self-doubt that she would really be good enough for the foster carer's environment. There was a hint of denigration of middle-class comfort and order and an idealisation of drunken squalor.

But there was nevertheless a reality-based issue of the strain of leaving one sort of world for another. It reminded me that even giving up hopelessness and dissipation is a loss, that hope and effort toward achievement are uncertain gains. There is some satisfaction, some peace, to be had in dissolute living.

Hannah: sexually and physically abused by parents

One problem, then, for young people whom we are supporting to break away from a cycle of hopelessness and failure is that they have readily available to them identifications in which they can easily shelter. 'No one in my family has even got a job, none of them have an education,' explained 15-year-old Hannah. 'I don't think you realise how hard it is for me to study.' Partly this was an expression of feeling that she could not rely on her family to help her in these goals, partly it was concern with betrayal of the family culture. But also in Hannah's case, as with Kelly, there was difficulty in believing that everyone has to work and struggle for achievement. Hannah, whose furious envy of other young people's achievements was always a feature of her sessions, expressed it as shown in the following extract:

> Hannah showed me proudly her prefect's badge which she explained the headmaster had given to her because she was more sensible than anyone else.
>
> 'He said I was trustworthy and would make a good prefect. I don't really know him – do you think he's just making me a prefect to sort of get me into the system, or just trying to make me feel better? This girl in one of the other classes, she was a prefect and she resigned or she had to resign – and I've been given the badge instead. I thought, well, I might as well do it . . .
>
> I've got so much work to do. I want to get enough GCSEs to go to college and I've decided I definitely do want to be a nursery nurse . . . I've got so much to catch up on, I have to work twice as hard as

> anyone else . . . And there's these smug bitches in my class who can just run around with their stuck up faces – probably learned it all in prep-school . . . and those little bastards Tina and Joey [younger fostered children in the same household], the whole house runs around them and what they need. How am I meant to study? I know what I'd like to do to them. I can't stand spoiled brats.'

Hannah's ambitions to work with children seemed sadly misplaced. The anger and venom Hannah expressed in relation to other children always pointed to her own feelings of need, of neglect, of having had too little in the past. She came from an appallingly abusive family where cruel punishments were meted out as a matter of course from sadistic parents. Her attachment needs for the parents and her conditioned fear of them prevented much anger or criticism being voiced toward them. Instead it was deflected onto her siblings and other children. In this session we can observe that children who receive parental care or teachers' approval are perceived as smug, spoiled, greedy and replete with knowledge or attention. Her own attempts to join 'the system' or to achieve GCSEs are full of the despair of having to catch up and work harder. There is also another factor that makes achievements the harder to work for, and this is indicated in the prefect's badge. Hannah has three conflicting versions of the reward given her by the headmaster: it may be a bribe to buy her loyalty, it may be an act of pity or it may be what someone else has thrown away, valueless. Although initially proud of the badge and telling me that she has deserved it because of being sensible and trustworthy, Hannah's distrust of authority makes her look for meaner motives.

Hannah's attempts to become educated and to secure a good future for herself were therefore ringed about with difficulties, not simply of an academic nature. Hannah's trust in adults was poor. Hannah's emotional needs were great. Her envy of other children was pronounced and led her to believe that they wanted to attack and denigrate her as she did them. Meanwhile, she easily lost faith in the value of her achievements. Later, we were to trace the difficult path from being a 'have not' to being a 'have'. If you have spent much of your emotional fury against achievers, how can you switch direction to become one of them? The problem of identification was a difficult one for Hannah.

In all of these struggles Hannah wrestled with an overwhelming sense of having nowhere to belong.

Her sense of dislocation was profound. She desperately wanted to go back to belong somewhere. Ironically, much of this sense of longing had been with her for years before she had been taken away from home – a fact she sometimes was in touch with but sometimes lost. Her need of her parents was so great that she was prepared to distort reality for them, to keep blame and anger away from them. Some of this attitude was trained into her by them because she risked their violence in any display of anger toward them. Like a hostage with violent kidnappers it was not safe to disagree with them. To hate and to be dependent on the person hated, to be brutally beaten and sexually used by parents on whom one has no choice but to rely: these conflicting feelings are the stuff of madness. It was intolerable for Hannah to let herself know as a child the full extent of her unjust situation. It helped her to believe that some sort of logic operated where she deserved her treatment. At least that meant that her parents were not arbitrarily persecutory. It also helped when she split the hatred between father and mother so that she found relief in hating one and siding with the other at times.

Hannah brought herself into care by 'telling' on her parents. The abusive situation of herself and her siblings immediately resulted in prosecution and imprisonment of the parents. And still Hannah longed to return. Once, after visiting her mother in prison, she confided to me that her mother had talked about the 'good times' they had had when she was little. Hannah had agreed and fondly told mum how she missed her. All the way home, Hannah told me, she had puzzled as to what her mother had meant about good times. In effect she could not bring to mind any good interactions between them, try as she might. 'Why did I agree with her then?' she asked me, and the answer came swiftly from herself: 'Because I'm too bloody afraid to disagree.'

It is probably only inmates of concentration camps or victims of torture and abuse who understand the reverence of victims for perpetrators. Even then, what fear can do to a developed adult personality falls far short of how it affects the developing child.

Hannah's capacity to hurt others was perhaps the most difficult legacy of identifying with abusive parents. The lie that the victim attracts their abuse, that victims are themselves to blame, was a lie that Hannah had made herself believe in childhood. It was the lie her parents forced upon her. Now that it could be Hannah's 'turn' to get rid of years of aggression and violence by inflicting it on others, her therapist constantly and annoyingly challenged this belief. Hannah often threatened to 'walk out and not come back' when I located aggression in her rather than her victims. In this way she revealed that the threat behind the lie was one of abandonment and disattachment. Her continual mistrust of me also constituted a hazard that threatened our relationship. She told me years later that she could not let me know how suspicious she had been of me. She could not believe people were really kind. 'I always thought you must be being sarcastic when you said nice things,' she confessed. As well as this being a reflection of Hannah's parents it was also because she knew her own behaviour masked her anger and hostility. When she had impulsively told her mother she missed her, for example, she hid her own anger and complaint. It was therefore difficult for her to believe I was not doing the same thing. It was four years before Hannah could reflect in this way with me.

Trust is not an intellectual exercise and I think it is only made possible by the constant repetition of an experience of being valued and respected. This is one of the reasons that therapy with abused young people is slow and cannot be hurried. A real alternative experience of an attachment is offered. The therapist keeps pointing to the reality of what is exchanged between herself and her client, seeking to convince, not by intellectual argument, but by pointing to the client's experience of the session. For example, young children who have been cuffed a lot flinch for some time before they stop this response in their sessions. These instinctive reactions are not really governed by the conscious mind. Even if the child keeps up a stream of hostile banter, their body is relaxing, learning from experience. Therapy has on its side the human being's capacity for reality, for growth, for adaptation to life. When I have witnessed the resilience and courage of so many of my battered clients I say to myself that, after all, even plants know to grow toward the light.

Jake – a 10-year-old boy with a mentally ill mother

Children who are beaten, neglected or abused seek to make sense of these experiences and inevitably keep some of the burden of blame for themselves. It seems that it is intolerable to most human beings to believe that they are the haphazard recipients of careless fate. It is easier to believe that hurt suffered was directed and pointed at the self. At least this latter belief establishes our importance instead of our insignificance. Children move gradually from an assumption that all events are motivated, to acceptance in maturity that only some events are personally targeted. It must therefore be a particular difficulty for children of mentally ill parents to discern the difficult conclusion that events are not necessarily motivated, despite the parents' claim that they are. I am thinking of parents who themselves believe that the world is organised along these principles. Particularly in paranoid illness the sufferer believes and acts on the tenet that they are being attacked. If the attackers are believed to be outside of the child and parent, the two are often merged in a nightmare experience where they fear the rest of the world. Instead of the child's finding relief and containment for his own fears he is instead flooded by psychotic anxieties from his mother. Then there are the moments, hours, days when mother believes he is the source of attack and she is vitriolic in her hatred of him. Fear of external attack makes him cling to her tightly. Vulnerable and afraid, he is suddenly derided and humiliated by her. A child in the arms of a paranoid mother is a child who learns that human exchanges can be the worst kind of nightmare.

I extrapolate these findings from the experiences I have had working with and supervising psychotherapeutic work with children whose mothers had major mental illness. The noticeable feature of their therapies was the quality of hatred that suddenly lashed across the room toward the therapist. Such experiences are difficult to convey. Being therapeutic means listening intently, dropping one's own guard to consider and think aloud about the feelings in the room. Therapists therefore have to be vulnerable to a certain extent, lending themselves to the process of feeling in a fairly open way. The experiences one has with children exposed to mental illness is an experience of sudden denigration, a nasty and wounding attack. It is not uncommon to find oneself full of hatred and fear toward the patient. The attack is often disowned so convincingly that it is common to think oneself unreasonably sensitive. Ashamed of one's feelings, one may cover up and pretend it has not happened.

Jake came into foster care and therapy when he was 10. He and his siblings had been 'educated at home' by his mentally unstable mother. She refused to believe that she had any mental illness, confounding the education services and social services for some years by claiming that she was living an 'alternative lifestyle'. The children were not allowed out of the house as gradually mother's paranoia took hold. They had months and years of living in darkened rooms with the furniture piled against the windows to repel intruders.

Jake had held onto a belief that his father, whom mother had banished from the house when Jake was 7, would return and make life better again. After a brief stay in a children's home before returning again to mother, Jake had told his social worker that he would like to see his father. This was completely against his mother's instructions to him and against her years of indoctrinating the children that their father was an emissary of evil. It took a year of once-weekly therapy to have Jake confide this experience to me:

> Jake was telling me about events when he was living with his mother. He said he had told his social worker when they were alone that he would like to see his father. His brother and sisters did not want to, or they wouldn't say so. No-one could ever realise how much guts it took for him to say it. He had thought about it a lot and he believed the social worker would have the power to arrange it. The social worker knew what his mother was like because she had been the one to get them out of the home with the police and all of that. Then she went and asked him in front of his mother, did he still want to see his dad and he had had enough guts to say 'yes'. Once the visit from the social worker was over, mum just went mad at him. She had screamed and ranted and raved. She had got hold of his hair and pulled him to the wall and hit his head against it until he agreed that he did not want to see his dad. She told him he was stupid, that there was a government plot against her, that the Prime Minister was ruining her life. Did he not see that all these people were spies, that social workers were government agents plotting against her? Their father was part of that plot. Was Jake also their agent?
>
> Jake struggled with this account and had to be reassured that social workers were not government agents in the way his mother claimed. He bitterly added that he and his siblings had no way of knowing who was right. His younger siblings believed that, as mother said, the postman was also sent to spy on them and they all had to hide when he delivered the letters. Jake felt humiliated now to realise his mother was 'lying'.
>
> His mother had made him phone up his social worker and tell her over the phone that he did not want to see his father . . .

This account is from a boy who was intelligent and mature enough to attempt to process some of these painful experiences. He was looking back with the benefit of hindsight and from the security that he would not return to his mother's care. But his emotional scars were often quite palpable in the therapy relationship with me.

In a session some time later:

> Jake tells me that he will be seeing his father tomorrow. I ask him what they will do together. 'You know what we're doing, I told you last week, don't you listen?' (This was said so venomously that I paused to collect myself.)
>
> 'I do remember that you were going to your grandparents' house . . .'

(Angry silence.) 'Well, now it seems that you are angry with me,' I say.

'No,' he replies. He is silent for many minutes.

'I seem to have turned into a careless non-listening therapist.'

He replies that he doesn't want to talk about it – let's change the subject. I say 'okay'.

Silence fills the room. I feel unnerved and unsure of how to proceed. I realise I feel extremely anxious.

'It seems to be difficult for us to talk today,' I say. There is no reply from him.

'Could it be that some angry or difficult feelings are getting in the way?' I venture.

'You said you'd change the subject and now you're coming at it just from another direction.'

'It's because I don't know what else to say: we seem to be stuck.'

'Then don't twist what I say! Oh, forget it.'

Uncomfortable exchanges like this peppered our sessions as the work went on and he became more confident. Initially I was open to the interpretation that they reflected my carelessness or lack of empathy. Gradually, however, I could feel that they amounted to a recurring theme of my inadequacy and my untrustworthiness. Jake was a very affectionate, sweet boy and his sudden venomous remarks which he refused to explore were all the more powerful because of the contrast. Then a long theme of anger and powerlessness at the hands of his foster mother became the focus of therapy. Many sessions were filled with angry tirades against foster mum. It was clear from these accounts that Jake allowed a lot of miscommunication between them without attempting to make his wishes plain. For example, he railed against foster mum's failure to fill in a form for him to join army cadets. He had neither reminded her nor communicated to her how important this was for him. He re-experienced impotent rage against a mother to whom he could not talk. When I suggested that perhaps a shadow of the past was falling on the present he was extremely thoughtful. He gradually began to acknowledge and to disentangle his real relationship with foster mother from the pattern of his relationship with his mother.

Whilst Jake became more open about his anger toward others he found it very difficult to acknowledge anger with me. Transference interpretations simply made him look terrified. He was so quickly persecuted and fearful of what may happen between us that it took a long time before we could bring these feelings into the open. After another fierce altercation when he accused me of forgetfulness, I addressed the subject of his fear of what my mind was like and whether it was a safe place to keep confidences. He immediately linked this to his mother's mind and his despair of communicating with her. He said that I could never understand what that felt like. Although I acknowledged the truth of this, I replied that I was being given a fragment of that feeling by the experience of his suddenly criticising and attacking me. I thought that my feelings on the receiving end, my fear and not knowing what to say were a replication of his own experience. At that moment he was like his mother and I was like Jake.

This interpretation had a strong effect on Jake. He had never realised that he could be identified with his mother and use similar vitriol. Yet, friends had told him that he could be very cutting and look very evil at times. He began to realise that he needed to be aware of this part of his behaviour, that he need not fear it to the extent that he felt 'mad like my mother' because it could be brought within the ordinary realm of control.

In this way Jake finally began to have the confidence to trust me and trust himself. It was never without reservation, however. He left therapy after two and a half years with a half-disclosure of sexual abuse by his mother. He decided he could not tell me all the details. It seemed important that he retain control over this confidence. His mother had continually told him that she knew his thoughts – they were her own. He perhaps needed to assure himself that I would not intrude into him, would respect his boundaries and his decision to stop therapy. He left on good terms, with a promise to return if he needed to in future. He remained with his foster family to maturity.

Identification with a parent is an everyday aspect of child development. When a parent has failed a child and is separated from them, identification may be fiercer and more necessary in terms of attachment needs. But identifying with a neglectful, abusive, drunken or mentally ill parent brings emotional difficulties right into the internal world of children. It is these internalised attitudes that can continue to disrupt the child's life. Therapy allows a focus on these inner turmoils which helps the young person to understand and control their responses.

Chapter 9

Restless children

Hyperkinetic disorder

- ADHD
- medication dilemmas
- anxiety
- emotional containment
- introjection of maternal object
- greeting cards in therapy
- joint working with colleagues
- hyper-vigilance or hyperactivity
- trans-racial placement
- self-soothing

Are children that appear inattentive, defiantly energetic, constantly active and restless suffering from attention deficit/hyperactivity disorder (ADHD)? (See Glossary.) Current child-psychiatric opinion maintains that it is useful to classify children on behavioural criteria alone. This means that there is no intended claim that ADHD has an organic basis or cause. This is not the case for hyperkinetic disorder which is a narrower diagnosis and requires the absence of other conditions such as anxiety states. Hyperkinetic disorder has a strong genetic component and is believed to be a brain disorder (Overmeyer and Taylor 1999). ADHD meanwhile is the mixed bag of difficult behaviour at home and school, in children who characteristically have multiple problems and complex histories.

The use of the term ADHD by the media and the public, however, suggests that children are born with a condition that is essentially meaningless and unpreventable, a biological disorder.

The major controversy concerning ADHD, however, is not its diagnosis but its treatment with stimulant medication, commonly Ritalin. Medication of an increasing number of active boys, on a behavioural basis alone, is a practice that stirs caution in many of us. Are these children suffering from a disorder or condition, or are they showing distress, poor attachment and deprivation? Have these children internalised an insufficiently containing parent and are they spinning with anxiety? What does it mean to medicate bad behaviour? What will be the longer-term consequences of medication? These are questions that bear particularly on children in public care whose experiences have been upsetting and whose behaviours are often extremely challenging. Seven-year-old Gabriel was just such a child.

Gabriel, 7 years

A learning-disabled boy in his third foster home, Gabriel was rapidly known by everyone in the Child and Adolescent Mental Health Service (CAMHS) where he came to see me. On arrival in the waiting room he would cycle round on the toddler's tricycle, shouting my name. He would kick on the door if I kept him waiting. When I opened the door he would shoot past me and run into and out of each room that had to be passed on the journey to my upstairs room. There were seven rooms *en route*. Grabbing pencils, overturning chairs, scribbling on paperwork if the rooms were empty, recoiling swiftly if the rooms were occupied, he would arrive at my room with myself in breathless pursuit. My colleagues seemed to enjoy my futile attempts to capture or control him. I understood completely what foster mother meant when she complained, 'He shows me up. I can't take him anywhere!'

I soon learned to take Gabriel firmly by the hand when I opened the door. I rewarded his compliance with brightly coloured stickers: one for coming straight to my room, one for returning straight to the waiting room. A special book in the waiting room was labelled 'For Gabriel Only' so that a few minutes could be spent with him finding it and, on good days, sitting down to look at it. Nevertheless, once in my consulting room, I found it necessary to alter completely my usual routine of letting the child choose which toys to play with and for how long. Early sessions showed an overexcited Gabriel opening one box of toys after another, distracted by another toy or idea before this one was set up or played with, whirling like a dervish from activity to activity. I learned to constrain him, therefore, to contain his impulsiveness by insisting he choose one thing at a time with which to play. Often I would make him sit on the floor and think and choose before he could get up and grab. Containment was a physical, concrete process as well as an emotional one. Acting as an adjunct to his weak sense of control and orientation I was able to help Gabriel regulate the boundaries of the sessions and contain a volatility which precluded his relating to me. In one session he had chosen 'painting' and settled quite well to putting large daubs of colour on the paper. He suddenly screamed an ear-piercing scream. He continued to paint. I meanwhile moved back in my chair. The scream had had an effect on me that made me wary; it had hurt my ears. Gabriel seemed unaware of both the scream and of its effect on me. This kind of incident happened several times per session. For example, in the middle of painting, the paintbrush whirled through the air and landed in a corner. 'Brush!' roared Gabriel. 'I think you can reach it,' I replied matter-of-factly, and Gabriel got down from his chair and retrieved it. He needed me to settle him back at the painting table, however, because once on the floor he glanced at the cars and wanted them. I began to see many of Gabriel's actions as not really volitional and full of meaning but quite the reverse. His actions were impulsive and opportunistic. He was carried along by fleeting pulses of interest that led to the next loudest stimulus to capture his attention. Both his attention and his intention were led by the incidental presence of items. His motivation seemed to be a passive recipient of his interest, not its master, I gradually concluded. The sudden screaming or throwing seemed to occupy his mind and attention for just as long as the action endured. For myself, reeling from the onslaught of these actions and trying to link them together, find meaning in them, anticipate their occurrence, I was treated as more or less an obstruction by Gabriel. He did not know why he threw the brush, he said; he did not know why he screamed, he just moved on hurriedly to the next thing. I concentrated on getting him to register that experience for me was linked, continuous, and could be thought about.

In his second session with me Gabriel pushed a length of string through the bottom of a paper cup. Whirling it above his head he spun around with it. Eventually the cup came loose from the string and flew off across the room. Leaping on the cup, he would have continued with this activity, but I limited him, saying he must be careful the cup did not hit me in the face. Defiantly he began again, but the cup immediately flew off, narrowly missing me. I showed him that we could tie a knot in the string to secure the cup and he continued for most of the session with this aimless but exciting whirling activity.

One day Gabriel chose to play with the train set. Having put the circular track together he loaded people onto the train, whisked them round and round and, once they had fallen off, he wanted to run off and play with the Lego. Trying to extend his concentration, I pretended that the little people were all jumping up and down saying, 'We fell off! What happened? Where's the train driver? Why did he make us fall off?' I assumed that Gabriel was the train driver and had the little people ask him what had happened. 'This is an express, a fast train,' he told them. 'It made us fall off. Why did we have to fall off?' I made them complain. Gabriel looked at me and sighed, 'I can't help it. I can't do it slowly. There's only one speed – fast. There must be something wrong with the train and it can't slow down.'

So Gabriel only had one speed, fast, and I began to feel sorry for the little boy caught in the middle of a body that cannot slow down. The moments were rare when interaction between us could be meaningful. I had to use enormous resources of energy to engage with him for an hour and I did not seem to be winning the battle.

My colleague, child psychiatrist Dr Ford, was supporting Gabriel's foster carers whilst I saw him. She performed an essential role in Gabriel's treatment, helping foster mother to understand the boy's problems and sympathising with the difficulty of the task. She also advised on strategies for managing Gabriel and emphasised that his cognitive and emotional age was nearer 3 than 7 years. We discussed the possibility that Gabriel was suffering from hyperkinetic disorder, a type of attention deficit/hyperactivity disorder. By this I understood us to mean that Gabriel could have a neuropsychiatric condition arising from a dysfunction in his body or brain. We were wondering whether Gabriel's defiant and oppositional behaviour was a result of his inability to slow down or attend. The kind of 'grab and run' naughtiness that Gabriel displayed granted him short-term rewards of attention and excitement. Perhaps he could not control himself enough for longer-term rewards. It could follow that his poor relationships with his carers and with his peers were a casualty of this necessity. The foster carer constantly spoke of him as if he 'would not', whereas it seemed likelier that he 'could not'. 'But he knows he's not to do that,' she constantly said. Yes, he knew, but was his impulse control sufficient to constrain his actions?

Dr Ford recommended that the foster mother and his class teacher complete behavioural monitoring forms, the Conners Rating Scales (1995), for two weeks. These forms comprise a checklist of behaviours as a daily record of a child's behaviour. (See example p. 141.) The same person(s) completes each set of observations in order that variation in the record is as much as possible a true reflection of the child's different behaviours. This scale attempts to monitor hyperactivity, attention and impulsivity. Gabriel's scores at home and at school fell very heavily within the 'very much' and 'pretty well' columns for most behaviours on most days. The pervasiveness of his disordered behaviour and its severity were marked. In this special school even the ratio of two adults to eight children could not contain him.

Of course, these data were simply evidence that Gabriel's impulsive, express-train behaviour was his common mode of being at home and at school. This does not rule out the possibility that deprivation or emotional turmoil was fuelling Gabriel's behaviour. Nor does it address aetiology, how the condition had been caused.

Observation	Not At All	Just a Little	Pretty Well	Very Much
1 Restless or overactive				
2 Excitable impulsive				
3 Disturbs other children				
4 Fails to finish things he starts, short attention span				
5 Constantly fidgeting				
6 Inattentive, easily distracted				
7 Demands must be met immediately, easily frustrated				
8 Cries often and easily				
9 Mood changes quickly and drastically				
10 Temper outbursts, explosive and unpredictable behaviour				

Gabriel's history

Gabriel's history was that he had been born to a mentally ill mother whose early handling of him had always required support. His records showed that he had always presented as a difficult-to-contain child, with developmental delay diagnosed at 2½ years.

He was noted as 'active and distractible' with delayed and disordered speech. He had received physiotherapy, speech therapy and occupational therapy, attending a day nursery and then a special school. His short attention span was often noted. Made a ward of court at birth, fostered for his first three months, then with his mother in a mother and baby unit, Gabriel's care was always shared with other carers. He left his mother when he was 5 years old and had been fostered since then, spending one and a half years with one family. He was six months into his second placement at age 7 when referred to me.

On the whole his history could be characterised as one of poor and disrupted attachments. But a thread ran through it of constant difficulties with containing or controlling his high level of activity. He was not perceived and did not present himself to me as a deeply worried, anxious, angry or distressed little boy.

My inclination was to judge that, however caused, his behaviour was hyperkinetic. It had a physiological flavour to it in that it did not seem to fluctuate with his emotions.

My psychiatric colleague, Dr Ford, diagnosed Gabriel as having attention deficit hyperactivity disorder and recommended a trial of methylphenidate (Ritalin).

The effects of the medication were dramatic. Gabriel became much more available, sociable and reciprocal immediately. He seemed happier in himself too, as if he felt less driven, less irritable in general. At school his teachers found him much more able to participate with his class, to learn and to gradually absorb skills. In therapy our first post-medication session was a much more pleasant and less strenuous affair. In the middle of playing a simple game he suddenly told me about his former foster carer, Susan, and her family. I talked about his missing her and he took this idea in as if it were new and interesting. He spoke of his birth mother for the first time and told me he was glad she visited him.

With Gabriel on medication the reciprocity possible in his therapy sessions was increased. He began to play simple games with me. He rolled a ball of string across the room to me and I rolled it back. He threw it to me, I threw it to him and we negotiated rules and game variations. On another day he wanted us to make a skipping rope out of lengths of string. The lengths he wanted were the size of the distance between us in our ball game. He wanted us to plait the strings together, but could not master the technique, nor did he want me to do it alone. Fastening the three ends of string to a desk drawer handle we wove ourselves over and under with string in our hands to plait the rope. Gabriel's pleasure in these joint activities was a joy to witness. I taught him the word 'cooperation' and we chatted about being a team and being together. What came alive in him was the possibility of a shared world, pleasure in communicating and understanding. Gabriel hated physical contact, which he seemed to associate with coercion and control. But he loved being on the other end of a rope from me. He often skipped, insisting that he and I turn the rope together despite the physical difficulty of this. He wanted to make a kite that he could take home in the holidays, and he did so.

I learned to offer my interpretations gently as ideas to which he may or may not relate. He was often desperate to control me, indeed to keep control of everything, and he reacted to my verbal skill with suspicion that I was nagging in order to control him or that I was demonstrating my superiority over him. 'Hey, Gabriel – when you are on that end of the string and I am on this end, we are joined up!' was likely to get a more thoughtful response from him than an observation that he wanted to be linked to me. But want to be linked to me he did. He wanted me accessible, close enough to be pulled nearer, far enough away for his own sense of autonomy. Gradually, nervously, with many displays of diffidence and contempt, he became nevertheless attached to me. Contempt was in his response to my Christmas card before the first break in our sessions. He opened the envelope, read the card, let it fall to the floor and proceeded to trample on it as he rushed to organise 'a very important game'.

I frequently give children greetings cards, which include the date on which sessions recommence. Whilst this practice can be interpreted as refusing to bear a negative transference I have not found it an undue impediment. To not return Christmas greetings from children seems to me heartless. When Gabriel returned from the breaks in therapy he was cool, diffident, careful not to betray any sense of happiness at our reunion. He avoided all but cursory glances at me. I found myself unsure, hurt, wondering did he really not miss me? This was a display of ambivalent attachment behaviour *par excellence*. The language of attachment, however, does not do it justice. The feelings evoked in me, in the countertransference, were the primitive child-feelings of wondering 'Does mother really love me?' Gabriel effectively provoked these feelings in me whilst he acted as a slightly bored, aloof visitor. At school, prior to his medication, Gabriel had learned very little and had tested his teachers to the limit. Now, with medication and therapy, he was more accessible and began to learn and acquire new skills. Nevertheless his teachers, like myself, found that underneath the hyperactive boy of the previous year, a poorly attached, troubled boy with anti-authority attitudes came into clearer focus.

In our sessions together I found that Gabriel lost completely his 'whirling dervish' activity. But he resumed it in an instant in my waiting room under the continuing critical gaze of his foster carer. Gabriel's carer was a plump, grandmotherly woman of similar Caribbean origins to Gabriel's own mother. She had heart and blood pressure problems. She lived alone, a single parent of many years. As well as Gabriel she fostered a younger extremely active boy and when he departed she took on the care of an infant of a few months of age. Despite her strictness and over-attention to good manners and tidiness she had undoubtedly invested a great deal in Gabriel in the two years he was with her. She had been responsible for instilling in him many patterns of behaviour that made him acceptable and liked by other adults. His table manners, his expressions of deference and respect when addressing adults, his good hygiene were all assets to a boy who had been likened to a wild animal on arrival. But 'Auntie Iris' found the task of containing Gabriel emotionally outside her capacity or comprehension. She felt that he was simply 'naughty' and unwilling to cooperate with her. It was easy, of course, for professionals like myself and the child psychiatrist to take a more benign view of Gabriel. We did not have to deal with his charged level of energy twenty-four hours a day. Iris perceived our efforts to help Gabriel as doomed to failure and, despite his improvements, he was unable to come up to her expectations. Gradually everything she said about him became negative. In the waiting room, when he produced a picture for her approval the sour response would be 'Well, you'll have to carry it home, I've enough to do.'

The situation sank from bad to worse. Gabriel began to refuse to go home at the end of his sessions. One day he lay on my floor and sobbed, 'Auntie Iris just wants me to watch television all day, it's boring, boring, boring! She doesn't like me.'

Dr Ford met fortnightly with Iris, trying to help her plan behavioural routines that might contain Gabriel. She had continually to emphasise his emotional needs which were those of a much younger child. Iris did seem to feel supported and listened to in these meetings and attended regularly. She experienced little support from the local authority, who had failed to enhance her payments despite Gabriel's level of difficulty, and had not organised any respite care. From her point of view, a short-term 'bridging' placement was lasting almost two years.

Local authority foster carers like Iris are given our most difficult children to look after without adequate training, support, remuneration or respite. Whilst Dr Ford was meeting with her the situation just about held together. But at the point that Dr Ford had to leave the clinic, Iris also gave notice that she wanted Gabriel moved. At that point he had been in therapy eleven months.

Gabriel reacted to these pending changes in therapy by becoming more controlling and challenging of me. Yet the strong connection between us forged in the early months was still evident.

An angry session immediately after my Easter holidays made me talk about his anger and disappointment that I kept going away. Three months earlier he would have denied this as he had done with my trampled-upon Christmas card. Now, however, he looked fiercely at my face and confessed, 'I didn't know if I was going to see you again until next Christmas!' Acknowledging his anger with me and finding that I did not reject him allowed him to continue to trust me with his feelings. As he became miserable with his situation at home, feeling he could never please Auntie Iris, he made a 'telephone' out of string and paper cups in his session. It was interesting for me to note the difference between the wild whirling of his cup on a string lasso during our second meeting and the use of the cup and string as a reciprocal connection between us nine months later. It was as if his capacity for attachment had been expressed as a wild lasso. Having found a relationship with me, it transformed to a telephone: a form of communicating across a distance.

Gabriel asked me to pretend to phone him and ask how he was. 'I'm still bored, doing nothing,' he told me bitterly. I noticed aloud how he wanted to keep his connection to me going across the distance of our being apart. I also voiced his frustration that I could not make things right for him at home.

During this period he left his sessions reluctantly, demanding extra time if he had been waiting and openly acknowledging that he liked coming to see me. It was a struggle for me to think how tantalising my strictly time-limited kindness must have felt.

In hope of finding foster carers who would better meet his needs, Dr Ford and I strongly advocated a two-parent family for Gabriel. We wrote reports stressing his need for physically active and emotionally containing adults. This was a very energetic 8-year-old boy. He needed parents who could channel his activity, a couple who could share his demands. He needed a father with whom he could kick a ball around, someone who could relate to his physicality without constantly quashing it. He also needed a level of resources that would enable a foster family to cope with his immaturity. He was not able to play out unsupervised, he was difficult in shops and on public transport, he woke early, did not sleep until late, and sometimes wet the bed. His demands for physical care were therefore strenuous.

West Indian couples wishing to foster long-term a child like Gabriel are rare. Gabriel was placed with another elderly single mother, Mrs Carter.

Another psychiatric colleague, Dr Moore, took over the supportive foster carer work with the new carer, Ivy. As Dr Ford had done, Dr Moore also supervised Gabriel's medication and monitored his weight and growth. In the early weeks Ritalin had made Gabriel lose his appetite and he had lost weight. This stabilised after a month but a close check was kept on this and other adverse reactions to the drug. Gabriel had monthly medical examinations as part of this careful monitoring.

Gabriel was very angry with his move of foster placement. He hardened himself to the loss of 'Auntie Iris', telling me, 'I don't care about her. I just don't care any more.' It was something of a relief to him when he finally left. He returned to his first therapy sessions after the move a sadder, more bitter child. In the following sequence we can see from my notes something of his responses to his loss just after the move:

> He made an angry entrance to the therapy room, complaining that he did not like my room and wanted the toys from the waiting room. He suddenly noticed some new additions to the Playmobil toys and rebuked me: 'Oh why did you get new things? Now there's too much.' He separates the new things from the old. He 'changes his mind' and is only going to play with new things now. 'The old things are rubbish.' He sets all the new toys up as 'a playground for children'. He becomes fascinated by the batteries in the toy flushing toilet. He claims they are wet and damaged. He wants to know 'which of the two batteries make it work'. He experiments, putting first one, then the other in. He is close to me now and lets me help him. I suggest he is like a scientist finding out about this. 'No, if I was a scientist my experiments might change people into a monster.' He lines up 'old people dolls' from the doll's house. He picks up a black mother doll and throws it viciously at the wall telling me to 'fucking shut up' when I start to comment. He gets angrier, dropping some figures and throws another. 'That's you, you're rubbish and I'm throwing you away.' I talk quietly about his wanting me to know what being dropped or thrown away feels like. He makes the people into a domino line and pushes them all down. I say he feels no one is safe. It's time for us to clear up and I say that this is hard but we have to finish for today in five minutes. He stops playing and begins to pick up all the toys. He drops one toy out of reach in the gap between my desk and the filing cabinet. 'I can do it, I can do it, don't help!' he commands. Bending in, he falls head-first into this hole, his legs in the air. 'Oh, no! Now you're in a hole and I'll just have to help you out,' I say, holding onto his legs. He is laughing and relaxes as I extricate him. He does not want to leave and continues to laugh and talk about falling in the hole. On the way out he reverts to behaviour I have not seen for eight months, running into every *en route* room in the building. I wait for him in the waiting room and when he joins me at last he says, 'I don't deserve a sticker today, can I come tomorrow?'

I hope that the level of intimacy and fondness contained in this meeting is communicated. Despite his angry entrance and the sudden rage when he swears and throws the mother doll, there is an undeniable connection and fondness between us. I think that the meaning of the session unfolds like this: Gabriel criticised me and my room as not good enough, preferring the waiting-room toys. He was swiftly conveying to me what he felt like when rejected as not good enough to remain with Iris. His perception of some new toys is coloured by this need to criticise and reject. It also gives him, fortuitously, an opportunity to grumble that new things spoil old things. This is a hint of the losses he has experienced by the new foster mother replacing the old foster mother. He deals with the change by claiming old things are rubbish. The old toy toilet, which he continues to like, he claims must be damaged. He explores how it works, seeming to resist the idea that things must work together to work at all. I do not realise the symbolism in this at the time but now it seems that it is a metaphor for Iris and himself. I pick up his wanting to find out like a scientist. There is a moment of genuine wonder as he lets me think with him about how things go right and how they break down. He voices his fear that he does not want to be so powerful that he could change people into a monster. Is this what he feels he has done with Auntie Iris? He seems fearful of his curiosity and anxious about people changing for the worse. At the same time I have not changed and he seems to be appreciative of this. Lining up the dolls he suddenly seems to be overwhelmed by anger. Is it Iris he throws viciously at the wall in his imagination? He quickly transfers this anger to me and tells me that I am thrown away like rubbish. All the people fall down, as if no one is safe. But Gabriel listens to me and seems relieved by my commentary. When he falls in the hole he lets me help him out. This is a little boy who usually does not let himself be touched. He seems enormously relieved to realise that I am able to help him. The replaying of his earlier chaotic behaviour now seems more of a message to communicate his disrupted state. Happily he agrees that he accepts my authority about sticker rewards and wants to see me tomorrow.

This session shows how ongoing therapy was able to bridge Gabriel from one foster placement to another and allow him to experience some continuity in the midst of chaos, some space to express his anger and fear, some hope to counteract his abandonment and rejection. Gabriel's treatment also indicates the viability of treating children in transition, provided therapy can be maintained across placements (Lanyado and Horne 1999).

During the next few weeks Gabriel attended his sessions with an increasingly hostile Mrs Carter. She found that he was difficult to control in the street and he 'showed her up' in church. It was difficult to help her understand that Gabriel was not really capable of sitting still in church and needed a tight system of rewards and sanctions for compliance in other situations – she felt he was simply naughty.

His behaviour at school also began to deteriorate. There was a request for an increase in his medication. After reviewing and monitoring his behaviour for some weeks a small increase and a different pattern of taking the medicine was recommended by Dr Moore.

Gabriel continued not to be a control problem within his therapy. However, he now often seemed edgy and snappy in our interactions. I noticed that he continually licked his lips and worked his mouth. When I had worked with amphetamine abusers many years ago these symptoms were understood to be a reaction to those drugs and I wondered at the similarity in Gabriel. Was his irritability an effect of his increasing misery in the foster placement or a side-effect of Ritalin? The drug that seemed to have opened a door to our relationship now felt like a barrier to my knowing him. Preoccupied and tetchy, he was often difficult to engage and I found myself relying on old games and patterns of interaction that soothed him rather than made him explosive.

ADHD: the research

Increasingly I wondered how far we were drawn into 'medicating distress in Gabriel'. The available research should throw some light on this issue as ADHD has been one of the most contentious issues in child psychiatry (Tannock 1998: 65–100). Nevertheless the critical questions have not been definitively answered. We are told that 'the core behavioural symptoms of inattention, impulsiveness and hyperactivity cause significant impairment in family and peer relationships, the ability to succeed in school during childhood and increase the risk for social isolation, serious driving accidents and additional psychopathology in adolescence and adulthood' (p. 65). So far so good. This tells us that troublesome children reported to have this spectrum of behaviours remain troubled and troublesome for many years. It does not tell us whether such symptoms have an organic basis or how they are caused. ADHD in North America is a heterogeneous condition, commonly diagnosed and under mounting criticism for the resulting medication of approximately 5 million children (Breggin 1997), an astonishing 11 per cent of the 6–17-year-olds in the population, 80–90 per cent of whom are boys. Critics of this trend highlight the multi-million-pound drug industry that benefits from it and question whether a generation of boys who commonly lack the presence of fathers is not being medicated out of its protestations (Widener 1998).

Reading Tannock's 1998 review one cannot fail to come away with a sense of caution, of partial and possibly erroneous directions in the search for understanding. For example, she writes: 'for the past two decades ADHD has been conceptualised as comprising three core clusters of behavioural symptoms: poor sustained attention, impulsiveness and hyperactivity (American Psychiatric Association 1980, 1987; World Health Organisation 1978, 1993)'. Some pages later she writes: 'moreover recent findings . . . challenge the construct validity of many dimensions of behaviour such as attention, hyperactivity, aggression and anxiety which have been assumed to be distinct (Hartman *et al.* 1997)'. This seems to be pointing out the risk of using muddled or variably defined terms which will contaminate the research findings and confound the attempt better to understand the condition. If ADHD is a poorly defined, vague and ambiguous set of overlapping symptoms, then we are unlikely to find discrete causes for it. I am overstating this pitfall, but twenty years of the term 'minimal brain dysfunction' being used in a similar way is a cautionary tale. Minimal brain dysfunction was discredited in the 1980s (Rutter 1982).

Whilst medication has been found helpful to a number of children diagnosed with these behaviours the research evidence is both a cautionary and a deficient tale. There is, scandalously, little longitudinal evidence of the effects of medication on children during their course of treatment. Responses to medication are not singular as Rosemary Tannock (1998: 67) summarises:

> [T]here is preliminary evidence that stimulant medication may not be as effective in reducing motoric activity in children with the aggressive type of ADHD compared to nonaggressive ADHD (Matier *et al.* 1992) 'highly anxious children with ADHD exhibit a less robust behavioural response and minimal or no improvements in working memory in comparison with a non-anxious ADHD group . . . [and] . . . are at greater risk for the side effects of stimulant medication (Du Paul *et al.* 1994, Pliszka 1989; Tannock *et al.* 1995; Urman *et al.* 1995).

These research caveats give substance to criticisms from opponents of methylphenidate prescriptions such as Dr Robert Furman (1996: 157) who states: 'Proponents of the diagnosis of ADHD . . . do not like to discuss the fact that the motor activity of almost anyone can be suppressed by psycho-stimulants (Rappaport *et al.* 1978) that there is firm evidence that the drugs do not produce any long-term academic improvement (Rie *et al.* 1976) and that the drugs may cause tics and interfere with growth'.

Child psychotherapists like Eileen Orford are pointing out that some of these children have not learned to trust, to wait, to contain their emotions in the sure sense that someone will come, will give, that their needs will be met. 'It does seem that what is effective with these children is help in organising the terrifying chaos of their inner worlds. (It is a terrifying chaos that has been with them since babyhood, which was not regulated at that time within the maternal environment and which has led to subsequent habitual and primitive responses of a hyperactive, hyper-vigilant kind)' (Orford 1998: 253).

Gabriel and increasing medication

And so back to Gabriel whom we did both medicate and give psychotherapy, the former allowing the latter at least to reach him effectively. It is as important, of course, to help Gabriel build resources and strategies within himself, to contain his emotions, however caused. A pill will not increase the child's understanding of himself, of others, of their effects on one another.

When further requests for increasing his medication were made, however, Dr Moore and I resisted this course of action. Gabriel had suffered the loss of his foster mother of two years, the loss of Dr Ford who gave him his medical checks, a change of class teacher, a change of social worker, and his current placement was under strain. It is worth noting in passing that there had been concern about the way in which his medication had been administered by Iris, with Gabriel claiming he was given extra pills for being 'extra naughty'. Even strict medical monitoring does not rule out the possibility of poor compliance with instructions and the effects of variability in doses.

In the six months he stayed with her, Gabriel and Mrs Carter's relationship exactly recapitulated the course of that of Gabriel and Iris. Within four months Mrs Carter gave notice that she wanted to have Gabriel moved.

Instead of increasing medication Dr Moore, Gabriel's social worker and I concentrated on getting him into a placement that could deal with Gabriel as he was. We jointly recommended a specialist fostering provision that provided its own school and therapists and supported foster carers. The carers who worked in this agency had access to twenty-four-hour social work support, ongoing training, enhanced payment and a supportive network of colleagues, family outings and respite care.

Ethnic issues for Gabriel

A further problem was encountered, however. This specialist foster care agency was in a part of England that had few Afro-Caribbeans and low numbers of black people. How should one weigh Gabriel's need for racial identity with his need for highly specialised provision of care?

Gabriel had experienced three foster homes with ethnically matched foster carers. The last two of these were with single black women of grandparent age, who had physical health problems, and both of whom had strong religious beliefs which inclined them to judge his behaviour as morally awry. They were, ironically, predictably unsuitable parents for a hyperactive, demanding, anti-authoritarian 7–8-year-old on every dimension save that of ethnicity.

American segregationist attitudes to race made popular through the influential Association of Black Social Workers and Allied Professionals (ABSWAP) have served to heighten our awareness of racial issues in foster placement. This movement may have been timely, ushering in an era of active campaigning for fostering amongst ethnic minorities. Nevertheless it did tend to replace evidence with ideology. Simon and Alstein (1977, 1981) produced longitudinal studies that showed satisfactory transracial placements were possible. Gaber and Aldridge (1994) presented strong evidence that black children were facing further disadvantage by waiting too long for racial fits that did not materialise. Meanwhile such children lingered damagingly in institutional or temporary settings.

Gabriel's need for a family that could contain him was judged a sufficient priority for ethnicity to take second place. His placement was jointly funded by Health, Education and Social Services: one of the rare miracles of bureaucratic liaison. In the event he was found a home with a black father, white mother and their two mixed-race children. In the strongly contained setting of the agency's school and the foster carers' supported home he quickly became an exuberant, energetic and remarkably happy boy. I visited him in his new school and he proudly showed me around. Since then I believe he has been doing very well and the plan was to see if he could be gradually withdrawn from his medication.

Funding of such placements is a perilous process and I have hardly dared discover whether Gabriel continued to be funded. Typically what happens three or four years on is that a financially strapped social services department decide that the cost of keeping a seemingly easy child in an expensive special provision is too high and the pressure to bring them to a cheaper 'in-borough' placement dictates a further move.

Jody: hyperactive or hyper-vigilant?

Not every child settles even in the supported setting I have just described. Jody was a little girl already using the maximum supported setting that a good specialised fostering agency can provide. She was 9 years of age when referred to me and already in her second foster home within the agency. Her current placement was under strain and the question was being raised, not for the first time, as to whether an institutional setting would suit her better. Jody's relationships with her carers were characterised by their perception of her superficiality, her treatment of people as interchangeable and her ruthless pursuit of material gains. Jody was a lively, chattering, wilful girl who was constantly flaring up with temper and irritability. She tried to boss everyone and bombarded her foster parents with demands. Her hyperactivity was of a restless, fidgety, not-able-to-wait kind. Fortunately she had saving graces. She was a pert, diminutive girl with a head of blond-brown curly hair and a pretty face. Something about her button nose, freckles and lively expression made her easily forgiven. She was an exasperating child. In the middle of a nasty attack, biting, pulling hair, roaring, spitting, screaming, she could be stopped in her tracks with the threat of a privilege being withdrawn. It was as if she thought mechanically, 'Oh yes, I'd like to go ice-skating tomorrow so I'd better stop this.' Like clockwork she could stop without emotion. The injured party, usually foster mother, bruised, bitten and upset, would find Jody's calculating coldness incomprehensible. A minute later Jody would be acting as if nothing had happened and seem genuinely unaware that the foster mother was upset. Jody's own upset was rare. Noisy displays of emotion for others had a feeling of falseness and could be switched on and off. She could, however, sometimes look lost, heavy with sadness and incomprehension. She was very aware that 'no one wanted her' but she was not reflective enough to understand why.

Jody's background was a chilling tale. She was the youngest of four children, all of whom had experienced severe sadistic sexual and physical abuse. The children had been brought into care without all the details being known. They had been helped to disclose their experiences by an experienced play therapist and a social worker. These two professionals saw the children together and let them discuss, show and play out their experiences over the best part of a year. These group sessions were frantically used by the children to play out their experiences of terror. All of the children had been beaten, tortured and sexually abused. It took several months for the legal case to be made against the perpetrators – their mother and her boyfriend – so that finally this couple lost their rights to visit the scared children.

They could not be contained in one family and each was eventually placed separately. At this point each child was given individual therapy.

Jody rarely mentioned her abuse to me although I had made clear at the beginning that I knew about it. Her therapist social worker worked closely with me in the agency and continued to play a part in supporting her foster carers. Jody seemed from the beginning pleased that the social worker and I continued to collaborate in her care. Jody's need for me to be a safe non-abusive adult was strengthened by my link to the social worker who had helped her and her siblings find protection and safety. Although it is an unusual pattern of work, the social worker's role in sorting out care arrangements for Jody, as well as having received the early disclosures, worked well in this instance. Of all the people to whom Jody half-heartedly related, her social worker was the nearest to an attachment. Jody trusted her.

My sessions with Jody therefore took place in a particular context of post-abuse work when she had been more than a year away from her mother's home.

The first few sessions taught me that, as with Gabriel, I would have to simplify the setting and minimise the number of distractions present in the room. Jody circled around the room taking out one toy after another, her play fitful and distracted, her wariness of me discernible, her restlessness constant.

Her play with the Plasticine was an example. Opening one pack after another she cut them into pieces. Later on she cut the pieces smaller. In later sessions the pieces were again cut. Reduced to fragments, Jody never made anything with her Plasticine until many months into her therapy I began to suggest we make things together. Usually I would make a basket or bowl and she would fill it with fragments. Months later she routinely played that the fragments were food and she would want me to be a little girl whose mother had put her in a room on her own 'to eat it all up and stop being naughty'.

Jody's sessions were filled with her non-stop chattering, controlling monologues. She was unable to use symbolic play and, like Charlotte, (Chapter 5) played out scenarios in which she assumed the personality of adults she had known, usually losing herself in the process. Most commonly she became an angry, preoccupied, hostile mother whose baby was a 'little bitch'. Over the months the personae of social workers and foster carers entered her repertoire and provided more benign characters than the resolutely punishing mother.

Although I saw Jody once-weekly for two years the major flavour of our meetings was of discontinuity. She rarely picked up a theme or activity from the week before. Of course, there was repetition of themes and activities, but there was little attempt to link one session with another. In effect she treated her sessions as separate entities and usually demanded to take out anything she had drawn or made. Each time I saw her she 'began again'. This experience of discontinuity was very pervasive and it is with disbelief that I see we had two full years together.

Jody came to her sessions pleased to be able to do what she chose and highly resistant to taking anything in from me. I gained some order in her sessions by applying the 'one activity at one time' rule, meaning that we had to put each game away before starting another. This device slowed down her restless tendency to get everything out and play with nothing. She treated most of my attempts to follow her as if I were trying to seize control from her. She would tell me to be quiet or brush my comments aside. It took many months for her not to automatically be persecuted by my autonomy. I resisted being allocated parts in her dramas except for short bursts of time. I would then declare that I was going to think about what we had played now. She regarded my thinking and talking with angry contempt and would repair to the sand tray and sulk.

Jody took in very little of my attempts at description or interpretation of her play. I realised that her whole approach to me in the room seemed designed resolutely to avoid noticing my autonomy. This could be considered autistic or as an indication of Asperger's syndrome (see Glossary) but it seemed to me more motivated than that. She did not present as autistic in the other spheres of her life at school or at home. However, she did test exceptionally poorly in terms of her intellectual ability, and her educational achievements were minimal. I thought of Jody's attitude toward me as one of keeping herself away and keeping me busy. She was mistrustful and very wary of me, suspicious of my intentions. Jody's whole pattern of relating seemed predicated on watchful determination to let nothing enter her except at her own request. Even words, looks and feelings seemed to be turned away before she could see their meaning.

I decided that I should not pursue my role of offering 'interpretation' to Jody. Instead I concentrated on helping her with another obvious series of difficulties. It was evident to me that Jody lacked the ability to self-regulate and this caused her particular pain when she was unable to self-soothe. So there were days when Jody came to her sessions telling me she had had a 'horrible morning' because another child had been picking on her. In an agitated state, everything she tried to do went wrong and her irritability showed itself in outbursts of rage at the paper, pens and me. I took an active part in recovering her from these states. She found it intolerable for me to talk about her despair, and when I had once tried this she had run out of the room refusing to return. Instead I treated her as I would a distressed baby. I helped with her drawing, I refused to let it be torn up as 'all wrong', and we drew a picture together. I determinedly praised her efforts, refused to believe she was 'rubbish'. I made declarations of faith that the Jody I knew was a really good artist and I liked what she had made. Gratefully she let herself be soothed and liked. By the end of the session she went back to school happy and recovered. Some days she came into sessions with a cold or having been sick, telling me she was 'poorly'. She did want her session, however. She made a little bed in my armchair and asked me to sing to her. I did so, partly to my own surprise, bringing to mind songs my parents had sung to me as a child. Jody loved these songs and learnt them. When she was upset from the news that she had to change foster placement she came in, made her bed, and sang to herself the appropriate 'I'm forever blowing bubbles', especially the line 'then like my dreams they fade and die'.

Perhaps this is not analytic psychotherapy. It is difficult to know if it was over-indulgent on my part. But ultimately it was about giving a child who has had too little of an experience of emotional containment, a little of this. I was teaching her too, how to soothe herself, comfort herself. I thought that in her case, instead of being an adjunct to her reflective and integrative parts of self, I was being a more basic, benign comforter, perhaps an adjunct to hope in the too-pervasive landscape of her despair.

I often wondered if Jody, who was undoubtedly hyperactive, would benefit from medication. When controlling oneself is such a difficult task is there simply not enough time to relate to others? She never was medicated as the social workers from her local authority were not in favour of it.

Unlike Gabriel's, Jody's attachment to me was strictly utilitarian. Because I made her feel better she came enthusiastically to see me. But on one occasion I had to miss her therapy because I was ill. When I returned I knew from experience that she was unlikely to show concern for me and might be annoyed that I had been unavailable. This was her usual attitude. To my surprise I was greeted with: 'Were you poorly last week? Are you still poorly?' I thought this was a sign of her real concern but my therapeutic caution made me respond: 'No, I'm better now, why do you ask?' 'Well, I don't want to catch it,' was the serious reply. 'You can catch being poorly, can't you?' Her words were a genuine attempt to grasp the nature of illness. She simply did not consider my feelings.

Jody broke down two further foster placements during the two years of her therapy. She remained a difficult burden for a foster family. For example, her very containing foster mother described how during their summer holiday at a Butlin's camp Jody had loved all the activities and contests. However, by the third day, families were actively avoiding sitting near them in the dining room. Jody, loud, bossy, energetic, would take over other children's games, sand castles, ice-creams. She was a liability in public places.

Trying to find better ways to help her, I read many articles about hyperactivity. A paper by Perry *et al.* (1995) about brainstem development gave me pause for thought.

The paper puts forward the hypothesis that because the brain is developing neural pathways in early infancy those connected with the trauma are laid down early on and as a basis for future development. This means that such children are over-sensitive to anything connected with the trauma and can develop into highly aroused, over-alarmed children.

Reading this paper I thought of Jody and of Charlotte and of other children who presented with such fixed, abiding difficulties in relationships and such marked hyperactivity. All of these children had experienced trauma very early on in their lives. Could their restlessness be more correctly thought of as hyper-vigilance? They are constantly fearful, constantly defensive, constantly on full alert. It is these attributes which make them so difficult to tolerate. They are exhausting to be with.

I am not sufficiently knowledgeable about biology to judge the neurophysiological arguments in this paper. But I do find the terms 'hyper-vigilant', 'over-sensitive' and 'alarmed' a set of accurate descriptions of a child like Jody. Indeed, it is not their activity levels that are the problem. It is their anxiety levels that wear us down. It is their attempts to control the world and escape any form of frightening control themselves which cause difficulties.

If Jody is a traumatised, alarmed child dissociating from relationships which have the threat of further trauma it is interesting to note that Perry *et al.* recommend as treatment: 'anything that can decrease the intensity and duration of the acute response or disassociation'.

It is no accident that I gave up interpreting Jody's alarm back to her. Instead I took it for granted and took the therapeutic task to be helping her to self-soothe and to engage with me in positive ways that enhanced her self-esteem.

Chapter 10

Trauma and its treatment

Post-traumatic stress disorder

- necessary caution in treatment
- multiply traumatised children
- identification with the aggressor
- defences of mistrust, denial, control and denigration
- traumatic memories during therapy
- double deprivation
- disorientation as a defence
- bullying and re-enactment of abuse
- trauma in the professionals
- conflicts acted out in the network
- therapy setting is crucial
- idealisation as a necessary angel
- ending and looking back

We owe a great deal in public awareness terms to the coining of the phrase 'post-traumatic stress disorder'. The American Psychiatric Association put this term on the map in 1980 and made publicly visible the clinical finding that human beings respond to traumatic events with a range of distressing symptoms. Over the decade 1986–95 the inclusion of children as PTSD sufferers was supported by overwhelming evidence (e.g. Yule *et al.* 1990).

Because PTSD has been defined it has proved possible and fruitful to research various aspects of these symptoms. In particular, work on memory and how traumatic events are recorded by traumatised people has opened an extremely valuable area of debate (Van der Kolk 1996). For many years clinicians had been describing traumatised adults who were dissociated from their painful experience. Instead of the expected responses of anger, hurt, fear, tearfulness, emotional upset, some patients seemed distant, flat, forgetful, cut off from emotion. Some seemed unwilling or unable to reflect on their experience and to integrate it with their other memories and their ordinary consciousness. Memories of the trauma seemed to have a life of their own from the sufferers' point of view. Instead of recalling events at will these patients described 'flashbacks' visited on them against their conscious control. 'Flashbacks' were not perceived as ordinary memories. Instead, victims described them as powerful, highly-charged fragments of the trauma scene which left the victim feeling shocked and shaken by the recall itself. These flashbacks may persist for the traumatised over months and years. Or they may disappear entirely after a few weeks. Other symptoms including anxiety, depression, panic attacks and phobic reactions are commonly involved and persistent following trauma (Green *et al.* 1994).

Defining these responses as a syndrome or disorder has given them much-needed credibility. Instead of the victim being allocated the burden of causation, instead of symptoms being attributed to the personality of the sufferer, the symptoms are relocated as an ordinary response to extraordinary events.

PTSD victims can claim dispensation from work, can be categorised as ill, can be legally compensated through the courts. These points are the good effects of a diagnosis of PTSD.

There are less good effects, however. Lumping all trauma into one category has led to generalisations which are not valid. If these generalised diagnoses are accompanied by a standardised treatment plan, as some proponents of exposure therapy favour, the results can be extremely harmful and painful to victims. Psychiatry and clinical psychology have strong traditions of generalising, quantifying, researching. Analytic psychotherapy has strong traditions of particularising, qualifying and working by case examples which are individual and *ad hoc*. Nevertheless analytic psychotherapists have had a wealth of experience in treating the traumatised. Attention to how the trauma is received and made into particular, personal meanings for the victim is as important in treatment as understanding that PTSD sufferers will carry an increased risk of anxiety disorders (Bolton *et al.* 2000: 513).

Children and young people in public care have inevitably suffered the trauma of separation from family. This is usually compounded by traumas experienced whilst at home, by their lack of access to safe, protective adults and by severe damage to their sense of trust. Some children have remarkable resilience to difficult experiences; others are overwhelmed by the duration or the number of traumas experienced. Some children's histories seem to be a catalogue of ongoing, compounded traumas barely separable from each other.

Treating multiply traumatised children is a different experience from treating an adult survivor of, for example, a train crash. The children I see have often no clear delineation of 'before' and 'after' the traumatic event.

Instead they have developed defences which blur and deny painful happenings: they use strategies of distraction, of minimisation, of manic cheerfulness or of placatory passivity. Some of these precautions are useful survival skills. Some become rigid defences which prevent good experiences getting through to the child. Because these children are out of touch with their experience it is often visited on others in a particularly nasty way: children who have been beaten can savagely attack a more vulnerable child or an adult at the point of vulnerability. Children who have been denigrated, sexually abused or scapegoated can be vicious bullies as they throw the unwanted experience into anyone who gets emotionally close. It can be a painful and hazardous process for a therapist contending with these reversed repetitions, on the receiving end of humiliating attacks on their own real vulnerabilities.

Matthew and the children's war

When Matthew was 5, social services intervened following a severe assault on the little boy by his father. Matthew had experienced several periods in care in the early years when his single mother could no longer cope with him, but from the age of 3 he had lived with his father. Both parents were young, involved with drugs and heavy drink. Matthew had lived in squats and 'bed and breakfasts' and any number of temporary addresses. His mother had abandoned him at 3 years and did not keep in contact. His father soon followed suit, so that Matthew had no links with his birth parents by the time he was adopted aged 8 after a further three years in a children's home.

Matthew was a clever, tough, challenging little boy who barely disguised his mistrust and contempt for adults and their authority. He created havoc and misery in his adoptive home and his embattled parents brought him, aged 9, for therapy to me.

Our early sessions were full of his highly defensive manoeuvres. He was cautious and secretive and seemed to make no concessions to my friendly attempts to understand him. He filled the sessions with games about aliens and weapons and elaborate fortifications. He took little trouble to explain the games to me. Tanks were the favourite means by which one set of opponents interacted with another. I talked about these highly defensive activities, emphasising the feelings of danger, of battle, of mistrust. I tried hard to attribute them to myself and him and his fear of encounter, his distrust of me. He routinely looked at me blankly and pointedly. 'No. It's just a game. It's a bit boring in here.' I was surprised by how defensive I felt at this criticism and felt a bond of sympathy for his adoptive parents. Indeed it was boring. An endless repetition of defensive talk and play with no apparent wish for real communication. He was so good at denigratory remarks that I often felt embarrassed by him, finding myself blushing at this derogatory attitude. At 9 years of age he could make me feel smaller than he was. Then one day he put aside the space wars temporarily, telling me I had nagged him to stop. He played with my doll's house for the first time and set up a family with parents and children inside. He then carefully placed a wild animal in each room. They were to be the 'guards'. Evidently they were to protect the family from attack 'from anyone who wants to break in and rob them'. Later he expanded this to 'if a boy was messing about in his room and his parents can't see him, the guards would get him'. One wild animal set on a wrongdoer and tore him to pieces.

Watching this play, it suddenly felt very graphic to me. Most of Matthew's sessions were intolerably dull, obsessive affairs with him endlessly adding layers of defences around his tanks and plotting hostile manoeuvres. He used mazes and maps and complicated codes. By contrast this little detail of a lion snarling and biting the 'messing' boy was alive and powerful. I suddenly remembered Matthew's own injuries at age 5 and, led by this thought, I asked him about his being mauled in the past.

He told me that his father just used to 'go mad' and would rain down blows on him whilst he desperately tried to curl up in a ball and keep his arms over his face. His father had picked him up and thrown him at the wall.

After he said this there was an instant of quiet which affected me deeply. It was as if the two of us now were witnessing the child and father suspended in time combined in attitudes of fury. We were the witnesses unable to intervene or help. It was as if I saw the boy hit the wall and slump to the floor. I had no words to help me and I fell silent. Matthew, however, became brisk and hurriedly went on with a complicated story in the doll's house.

This little fragment of trauma seemed to be suddenly detached from Matthew's cool evasive way of relating. He would not, however, tolerate much discussion of it or allusion back to it. Instead he showed me that children and adults were involved in an ongoing 'war' in his games. The children wanted to take over the house and playground for themselves. The adults wanted to control them. In his play the children barricaded themselves behind slides and swings and turned the roundabout into a clever weapon. They looted the home for treasure.

Matthew did allow me eventually to link his deep distrust of adults to his early experiences. The brutality that he had experienced was linked in his own mind with occasions when he lost his temper and punched, kicked and tore at his adoptive carers. At these moments he seemed to shift from rage that they were saying 'no' to him, to an enactment of brutal uncontrolled aggression. He admitted that he was not sure at some points who was hitting whom. Although he was doing the punching he was overtaken by a vendetta against frustrating adults and his satisfaction in his own power was something he found hard to condemn. He would not accept the fact that he was becoming the bully that he hated. In his mind he needed his defences, he needed his protective rages, he needed to feel in control, he needed to use powerful aggression. The consequences of these defences for his relationships was a price Matthew seemed prepared to pay. He consistently complained at having to see me, he constantly told his adoptive parents it was a waste of time.

In his case, broken and disturbed attachments made the impact of a traumatic beating an abiding grudge that Matthew nursed against the authority of adults. Gianna Henry (1974) called this defensive stance 'doubly deprived' because an original state of deprivation is responded to with defences that further deprive the child of good experiences.

The experience of trauma fragments, toxic and powerful, which shoot into the receptive therapist is one of the hazards of this work. I say this because such experiences stay with you and sadden and burden the recipient as well as adding to one's understanding. I have learned therefore to be cautious and respectful of my patients' reluctance to tell or to revisit emotionally traumatic events. These happenings are hard to bear even at second-hand. In Matthew's case my feelings were heightened by his eventual withdrawal from therapy, leaving me with the pain of not being able to help him. Whether the transference of this helplessness relieved him at all remained unclear. He stayed with his adoptive parents, however, and they struggled to manage his marginally improved behaviour.

Alan: a 'shell-shocked' boy

Eleven-year-old Alan had been through a catalogue of neglectful and abusive experiences. His young mother, unable adequately to protect herself, was simply incapable of parenting him. She loved him, however, and continued to visit and be visited by him through all the difficulties of his foster placements from the age of 7 onwards. For his part he was fiercely loyal and fondly attached to his mother. All of Alan's abuse had been at the hands of mother's boyfriends and partners. One incident that kept returning again and again to haunt Alan was when his arm was broken and he was not taken to hospital until the next day. He had become confused, in shock by the time of his arrival at the hospital.

Whereas Matthew had developed harsh interpersonal defences to protect himself, Alan seemed to have no defences. He shook when confronted with a question. He lost his way to my room for many sessions after we had begun regular therapy. He presented himself as a pale, thin, nervous boy who could barely hold himself together. Bad experiences had made him forgetful, confused, dazed. With his ashen face, his stammering manner, and his shy anxious demeanour, Alan looked shell-shocked.

It was only gradually that I began to realise that, as well as being a reaction to stress, Alan's disorientation had a defensive quality. Sometimes Alan could be very astute and his shell-shocked manner could be used as a cover for his non-compliance. Underneath this apparently placatory attitude Alan was wary and sometimes very controlling, coming late and leaving sessions early, engaging with me, it seemed, on his own terms.

His fear of me was real, however, and I had to suggest very cautiously some of his less obvious motives. Alan had a difficult time with his peers and was often the target of cruel jokes and bullying. What was less apparent at first was that he invited attack. This seemed to be a replication of his own abuse and he made constant loud appeals for rescue by an adult. Alan seemed to be in need of continual reassurance that adults would intervene to help him. He viewed with great suspicion, however, their attempts to do this. He filled me with tales of his school teacher's sadism. Whilst aspects of this may have been true there was a sense of relish and satisfaction that they were bullies. Alan's own bullying was performed on the family pets and he could not be left unsupervised.

Gradually Alan acknowledged some of his own aggression and anger. He was greatly relieved at my tolerance of these nasty aspects of himself. I helped him distinguish between angry feelings which cannot be helped and aggressive actions which can be controlled. As Alan took back into himself his own anger and aggression he seemed visibly to put on weight in front of me. He became more substantial and less of a waif. Now it was only when upset that he became disorientated and confused. Gradually he managed to deal with these defensive strategies as well, at least recognising them. 'I'm in a state aren't I?' he would say. 'I may be able to talk about it when I've calmed down.' Alan frequently used me as a target for his grief, accusing 'therapy' of upsetting him. As he made a very convincing victim I was once desperate enough to retort that I did not force him to come and he could stop if he wanted to. After fifteen minutes of 'Well, that's what I'll do then, stop coming,' I still had not argued with him. He finished lamely: 'Look, you know I only say that because I'm upset.'

Alan struggled with reality, often taking cover for long periods in compensatory fantasy. He could convince himself he was a famous footballer, that everyone adored him and wanted his autograph. Derailing his mind from unpleasant reality had become a defensive manoeuvre that was at his disposal for current stresses and strains.

He continued to be haunted by the trauma of breaking his arm, reporting to me dreams in which he broke his arm at school and ran away. In the dreams his teachers chased him to bring him back to his lessons. The hurt, traumatised boy could not seem to grasp wholly that there were friendlier more protective adults available now. Alan nevertheless made a good relationship to me and maintained his therapy for three years. As well as helping him link past events to current fears, I tried to amplify his 'small voice of discontent' so that he could more clearly put his own viewpoint. He became more assertive as he matured, even chairing his own Child in Care Review on one occasion. He was pleased that he managed to see more of his mother by challenging cancelled visits. He remained annoyed that after breaks in our sessions I would not see him for two or three hours to compensate. In our relationship he became able coherently to present his grievances and demand for compensation.

Aged 14½ Alan's improvement was noticeable to his carers and teachers alike, and it was with some satisfaction as well as sadness that we said our goodbyes. A year later I visited him, and was struck by his physical growth and easy conversation with me. He was rather an isolated young man, however, and there were still concerns about his future prospects.

Simone and traumatising therapy

Simone was a child who seemed desperately in need of therapeutic help but the process could not be sufficiently contained to benefit her.

I first saw Simone with her brother and sister when she was nearly 5, following their father's imprisonment for sexually abusing a neighbour's children. He voluntarily confessed that he had routinely sexually abused his own children as well. Simone's mother would not accept the fact of their abuse and, when she did so, would then not admit that it had affected them. She remained loyal to the children's father. Their mother gave the children contradictory and confused messages according to the pressure on her to acknowledge their abuse. She gave the children no permission to reveal details of the abuse and actively sought to silence them and renew their links to their paedophilic father. Thus, despite explicit instructions to the contrary, she smuggled in gifts and cards 'from daddy, with love'. She seemed not to notice how still and fearful the children were at any mention of his name. The children made clear to everyone that they did not want to see daddy. They did want to see mummy, however, and it was tragic to hear mother constantly refer to their reconciliation when daddy had served his sentence.

Eventually, after two years of such fortnightly visits, the children were protected from this repetitively painful scenario. Visiting contact was severed and they were confirmed in their placement for long-term foster care. After a further year in placement Simone was referred back to me for ongoing therapy. She had developed into a hard, smart, challenging little girl of 7½ years. She remembered my earlier interviews when she had confided in me that her mother had known about and participated in their sexual abuse. Simone was ambivalent about seeing me regularly but her foster carers and teachers were having great difficulty containing her. She could work up into a mood of tantrums and hostility over the course of a day, 'like a storm brewing' said the foster carers. Her behaviour could be extreme: she had smashed windows and set fire to her sister's bed. At night she would roam the house and steal all the sweet things she could find in the larder and fridge. The foster carers became very vigilant and controlling to manage Simone. By contrast, her school perceived her as a 'poor thing' and gave her extra time and attention readily. They called the foster carers to retrieve her when she became unmanageable. The school and foster carers became critical of each other, tending to split the unintegrated behaviour of Simone into 'simply a distressed child' and 'simply a manipulative child'. This sort of split is a common hazard of adults struggling to deal with difficult and deeply ambivalent behaviour. In effect it is necessary that the adults realise that children like Simone are not 'either-or' but 'also-and'. That is, Simone was a distressed and manipulative child, hurt and angry, waging a vendetta against adult control because she could not trust adults. It would have been of enormous benefit to Simone if the adults could have responded to both parts of her, kept in mind both parts of her, as they dealt with her. Unfortunately this was only partially the case, and both school and foster carers continued to play out Simone's ambivalence for her. When at school, Simone portrayed her foster carers as strict and aggressive, a characterisation that some staff seemed very happy to believe. Meanwhile she carried home tales of how she had been allowed to stay in the head teacher's office and not do the maths she disliked. She openly smirked during these reports.

In her therapy, at least, I strove for an integrated view of Simone. She began to arrive at my consulting room and burst into floods of tears. Somehow through the sobs she managed to ask for a drink and a chocolate bar. I gave her a drink but not chocolate. In my room she suggested that I give her gifts of paints and Plasticine and was quick to assume that I had selfish motives for not doing so. She was genuinely fearful of me as well, the gifts being needed perhaps to concretise my good intentions toward her. She followed this by giving me gifts of her drawings and paper models, telling me fiercely to take them home with me but not to let 'your daddy see them'.

I began regular sessions with Simone in February and we had only four meetings before the Easter holiday intervened. When she returned after a two-week break she was noticeably more reticent and tentative. The following week she brought with her a doll given to her by her mother. She cried piteously, saying she did not want to stay with me. She said she hated coming to this building because she used to see her mother here. This was true, as the therapy rooms and access rooms were part of a specialist centre. No amount of gentle talking could calm Simone and she worked herself up to hysterical sobbing. I took her out early, trying to reassure her that it was all right to bring these painful feelings to me, but I would be trying to not let them overwhelm her. There followed sessions in which a crying, reluctant Simone would take twenty minutes or so to come upstairs to my room. Her school escort looked at me as if I were someone to be feared. The school let me know that it was becoming impossible to get into the taxi with her. I arranged for her foster mother to bring her and I tried sessions with the two of them. It was useful having foster mother there because she explained to me that Simone very much associated seeing me with seeing her birth mother. Simone had often cried at these visits and at her mother. She had been routinely placated with sweets. We were able to talk openly about how confusing and upsetting it was that I should be associated with the same place where the visits occurred. I was also a professional who had agreed that Simone needed protecting from her mother. Simone was able to say she would prefer to see me somewhere else. Sadly this was an impossible alternative for me. We managed with foster mother's help in escorting her to continue the sessions productively until the summer holiday. Simone's sessions at this time were an interesting mixture. She showed me her cuts and bruises from various incidents. She told me she had stolen her foster mother's necklace and took in astutely that I would not 'tell on her'. Fortunately it was an inexpensive one so I had not too many qualms of conscience that my role was to interpret her motives and the repercussions on her relationship with her foster mum. She was quick to limit and control me and then to ask reflectively if she was bossy? Her friend had said she was. I replied that she may want to control me because the alternative was that she must trust me. She would need to believe that I would not hurt her with my independence. Simone was a clever 7½-year-old and she took this in gravely. A little later she said, 'I like you but I'd also like to punch you.' I replied that I could understand her feelings but that I also would not allow her to hit me. She looked at me approvingly so that I had to smile. Her combativeness was an aspect of her I automatically appreciated.

When the summer holidays intervened I cursed my bad timing in beginning therapy when I had, before Easter. I could feel the nervousness with which she left her last session before a six-week gap, Sellotaping her box fiercely 'to keep the others out of it'. I judged her engagement with me to be tenuous.

To my surprise, she returned in September quite composed and came to my room without a murmur. She soon showed me that she had a computer pet with her and taught me how to play with it. After ten minutes or so she said obliquely that it was all right for us to play with it 'because she would get it back to Sean's room before he came home from school'. So I had become an unwitting accomplice to theft and I shook my head trying to choose my words carefully so as not to insult her: 'Oh, so this is something that you have taken, borrowed, without Sean knowing and now you have us both playing with it!' 'Yes, I am a thief,' she agreed happily. The session ended with us negotiating the rules that she could not take her drawings home but she could show them to her foster mum at the end of our time together. I had decided that I would enforce this rule about 'therapy things staying in the therapy room' to emphasise the boundary between the session and the rest of her activities. As it had also a meaning for her about who controlled the session I felt that she would ultimately feel safer if I continued to emphasise my control. I could feel both her respect and her determination to be a match for me.

The following session found her busily involved in making a rabbit out of paper. She was insistent that I take it home with me. There was a shrewd test mixed in with this insistence. I let her know that it was best that neither of us took the things she made out of the room. 'Would your daddy see it?' she asked, suddenly anxious. 'Hide it in a drawer,' she urged me. 'Put it under the other things and he won't see it.' It was the end of the session and I felt she did not absorb my response to this, which was along the lines that she was assuming my home was like hers had been with her mother.

Four weeks later, Simone's foster carer again came to see me. She explained that therapy sessions were having an extremely disruptive effect on Simone. The day before therapy Simone would be anticipating seeing me and become disruptive and unable to work at school. On the day of therapy she was excited and tense, unable to concentrate but simply waiting for the session. The day afterwards she was remote, thoughtful and easily flew into a rage. The school staff were asking for therapy to stop. Foster mother was having to remove a distraught child from the school when she became unmanageable.

My fostering agency colleague and I tried in vain to address these difficulties in meetings with school and local authority social workers. School staff regarded my work with deep suspicion and further differences emerged between them and the fostering agency that employed me. The local authority social work department had been reorganised and a new set of social workers came to these meetings. They soon began to question the children's placement, fuelled by doubts about the foster carers amongst the teaching staff. The children's birth mother relentlessly campaigned for access to Simone and her siblings. At times, the newly allocated social workers seemed to forget the extensive nature of the abuse suffered by Simone and took her poor behaviour as evidence of poor foster care. They questioned the 'brutality' of mother's lack of access. The two years when Simone had continued fortnightly to have access to a mother who talked fondly of her abusive partner and was openly defiant of the Child Protection Plan were considered insignificant in Simone's current behaviour.

In this situation my own need for supervision was more than clear. Child psychotherapists, however experienced, usually have regular supervision and my then supervisor, Monica Lanyado, and I talked the situation over many times. We were both inclined to the conclusion that therapy in this atmosphere of distrust was impossible. The added difficulty of the therapeutic setting being for Simone so inextricably bound up with her mother's visits, further loaded the strained sessions. When Simone actually was with me she could gain some comfort from my real presence but before and after the sessions I think she was plagued by uncontainable fears. Instead of the adults forming a strong and confident team around her, the adults were suspicious of each other and undermined each other's work with Simone, a situation of which she was undoubtedly aware.

I decided to respond to the qualms of the network by suspending Simone's sessions for three weeks and monitoring her reactions. When I explained this decision to Simone with her foster mother present Simone immediately protested that she wanted to keep coming because she liked therapy. I outlined her difficult behaviour at school before and after sessions and expressed the view that therapy must be careful not to stir everything up in her so that she is too distressed to manage. Her foster mother waited downstairs whilst we had a final session before the three-week break.

Simone told me about all the special treats she received on her therapy day like being able to choose a friend with whom to have an early lunch in order to come to see me. She played busily as we chatted. She built a castle with thick walls, using a box of bricks. Thieves came to the castle to steal the treasure, she told me, and they loaded it all into a van. Nobody knew they were stealing because they were clever actors. Gradually they stole the entire castle, brick by brick. I wondered aloud whether Simone herself was the thief, referring to her earlier self-description, or whether she was feeling she had been robbed of therapy by me or all the clever-acting adults. She began to loudly declaim that past thefts were a mistake, 'I never took Vivian's necklace . . .', until I gently said why should she trust the grown-ups to give her things when she had not been given what she needed? It may feel safer to be secretive because, if you really trusted and needed someone, what if they let you down? What if I was not to be trusted, how would she know? What if I did not help? She gave me one of her acute looks, falling silent.

'Let's hide all the treasure over here,' she said. 'We'll sort it out another day.' I said that Simone was showing me that she felt that there was something valuable in therapy that she was putting away for now, and I helped store the bricks in the cupboard.

She now turned her attention to the baby doll, handling it roughly and playing a game where the baby fell from the chair, then out of the cot, and Simone, as mother, rebuked her, saying it was her own fault because she was messing about. Instinctively I defended the baby, saying that really a mum has to be responsible for the baby and make sure she cannot hurt herself. She said suddenly, 'Is it a two-year-old's fault if she hurts herself?' She explained that, at 2, she and her 1-year-old brother had pulled the bookcase down on top of themselves. 'It must have been mummy's fault then for leaving us alone,' she said grimly. She asked me about another incident when she had fallen and cut her head, then another where she got lost in a shopping centre, and a string of other events came tumbling out. I talked about her seeing me reawakening memories of many hurts and worries she had experienced with mummy. She seemed to want to know if it was her fault that she was not kept safe. Also in our session at that moment she may be wondering why could I not have kept her safely in her therapy. Was it her fault for messing about? I emphasised that it was indeed my responsibility and I was not blaming her for ending therapy. She gravely asked whether she could come back and I responded that we would see how she felt about it when we next met. She gave me instructions to look after the baby doll very well when she was away. 'Don't leave it here,' she urged. 'You should take her home with you.' Before parting she fixed me with her beseeching look and started, 'I like therapy and I like being fostered with Vivian.'

Following this session, Simone's behaviour did calm considerably. She no longer had to be removed from class. When I met her with foster mum, Vivian, three weeks later, we discussed openly Simone's need for help but her difficulties in using it. Simone volunteered that it was the building itself she hated: she would like to have therapy with me elsewhere. Sadly I could not arrange this and I had to content myself with a strong recommendation for Simone to see another therapist in a different setting. The social services department was unable to arrange this. Although a break in treatment was probably of benefit, I remained concerned at her needs being so neglected.

This experience made me deeply aware of the tendency of networks around a traumatised child to re-enact aspects of the trauma. Simone split her own knowledge of abuse and colluded with whichever adult was present, pushing blame and mistrust out to the non-present adults. Unwittingly, this behaviour was repeated by the adults, setting them at odds with each other. It is a frequent occurrence with such cases that members of the network seem to forget the reality of the abusive experiences encapsulated in the child. A 7-year-old child is therefore able to divide and rule the adults. Ironically it is often the case that the abusive parent, full of denial of their own actions, begins to be perceived by social workers as a safer haven in the storm of network conflicts.

For my part, I wryly perceive my blindness to the toxicity of a therapy setting where fraught access visits with her mother were carried out for far too long. Simone herself felt the setting was impossible. Perhaps I was unwittingly drawn into a re-enactment drama of her separation from mother. If so, I hope it was a re-enactment that brought her some relief.

William

The theme of repetition of an abusive or traumatic scenario is one I have become used to in the therapy room. It is, of course, part of the usual pattern of therapy that the patient transfers to the therapist experiences of relationships in the past. However, with traumatic experiences, this transference is of a particular quality. Sometimes, as with Matthew

(p. 160), there is a sudden heightening of experience in a seemingly banal interchange. Receiving these communications is to be suddenly filled with dread or alarm or experience of an uncomfortably vivid kind. The experience is one of finding one's own defences bypassed or shattered, even if it is for an instant. The experience can feel like having some hard, bright shard of pain swiftly deposited into oneself.

William, a boy who came for therapy for six years through a long career in three different foster homes between 10 and 16 years, was another cut-off, deeply damaged boy whose mother had beaten and scapegoated him mercilessly. William always came for his sessions, was obliging, tentative, placatory and found it hard to know what to do with the time. Something in his manner made me endlessly patient with him. I knew that he liked me, that he wanted to trust me, that these silent, awkward sessions were his best effort. For my part I held a strong belief that he would be alright, that he would manage to keep himself on a path to recovery and to development through all the vicissitudes of school suspensions, fostering breakdown and minor delinquency. I found it no effort to have faith in him. I sometimes challenged myself that we were mutually idealising but if it were so like the necessary angel (Alvarez 1992: 118) I could not persuade myself that it was destructive.

An air of boredom and inactivity was pervasive in William's early sessions but it had a gentle, longing quality to it. William quietly made a board game – snakes and ladders – when I replied to his enquiring that I did not have such games in the room. I think he understood me to mean I lacked them whereas I had meant that they were not useful. I had not the heart to refuse to play, however, when weeks of careful toiling had produced a good-enough substitute. We played several games and I found myself puzzled as to how easily I broke my own rules to play frequently with him. This was hardly therapy, I criticised myself, reminding my conscience that I was paid to help and heal. Fortunately this was before the days when insistent demands for measurable outcomes were in vogue. I had no measure of the helpfulness of this activity to William other than his regular early arrival, his habitual air of world-weariness gently lifting through the sessions and his exit with a happier air. Some games he won, some games I won. I tried hard to seek the meaning in these games: 'You keep the rules, you are very fair,' I said, amongst other things. 'So do you,' he replied, and then, 'not like my mum'. Haltingly he told me that his mother played computer games and she would always beat him. After a pause he told me in a flat voice about other types of beating she gave him. The stories were truly horrific so that I even wished he would stop telling me. His humiliation at her hands, his silent judgement of her unfairness was released at that moment. His sessions returned to their quiet activities. Months later, another fragment of his story came out. His mother had held him under the water in his bath. More quiet sessions followed. Then another shard of horrific memory. It was three years before he let me know that he was haunted by flashbacks of his being beaten at home. Sometimes his mother had dragged him out of bed and sleep to hit him. These memories came out in fragments so sharp, so cutting, that we needed the gentle intervening sessions to recover.

William taught me that recovery from many years of abuse takes time and care and cannot be hurriedly achieved. Memories of overwhelming pain are in themselves painful. I was glad that I was patient enough to follow, to let him lead me to the events he needed to revisit. At 16 he ended therapy, though he visited me from time to time. William grew into an 18-year-old college-attending young man. He brought his first steady girlfriend to meet me. He attributed much more retrospective insight to me than I actually had had at the time. He had frequently, he said, had to contend with flashbacks before the sessions but could not always tell me about them and did not want me to talk about them. He felt that I knew anyway and that he always felt better after the sessions.

Some children like William do not transfer the relationship of the past onto the therapist. William was acutely aware of my difference from his abusive mother. His therapy with me was an opportunity for a different, fairer and more pleasant relationship.

As a therapist one fights against sentimentality and fictionally happy endings. Real therapy is a ragbag of loose ends and unanswered questions and uncertain outcomes as well as satisfying shared and completed work. Nevertheless I feel that as well as the grief and the pain of therapy, as well as the bafflement and boredom, it is an unending privilege to have been a part of children's life stories.

Epilogue

Adaptation of technique

– interpretations in positive mode
– destructive defences
– joint working
– long-term therapy
– weekly and twice-weekly therapy
– a child's capacity for linking
– lost and found

In this book I have sought to make the general point that children who have suffered losses, neglect and abuse may need a therapist to be particularly aware of their external situation, past and present. Therapists may need to adapt techniques that are based on the treatment of children in more or less functional birth families. For example, children who have encountered hostile and abusive adults may need a therapist to be extra communicative and receptive as the quietness of a therapy room may overwhelm the child who dreads being persecuted. This is no more than ordinary atunement of therapist to client, but it relies heavily on a therapist's awareness of experiences on the edge of being unbearable. For example, a young woman began her therapy with me by suddenly leaving the room after fifteen minutes, returning five minutes later and leaving before the end of the offered time. Several sessions of a similar kind followed this tentative start. Despite a 'cover story' where she would seem to take offence at something I said, it was eventually clear to me that she felt impelled to leave the room to keep our engagement under her own control and to avoid her feelings of claustrophobia. She told me much later that often she had been locked in the bedroom with her abuser. Interpretation of her fear of me had to wait until she could master it enough to take in my words. Initially her need in the room was to avoid my putting anything at all into her. Simple patient reassurance may be a necessary prelude to conversations that reveal feelings or fears. Therapists may need to hold onto what they feel for a longer time before they can offer it back as insight.

When a child is in foster care, removed from their birth mother, interpretations with the word 'mother' in them can be particularly tricky.

Talk of 'a therapy mother' or parallels from child and mother to child and therapist may deeply wound and be misunderstood. To seem to claim that missing a therapist during a summer holiday is equivalent to missing an absent mother is insulting. The interpretation needs to be phrased as missing the therapist reminds the child of missing mother and confirms in the child a feeling that grown-ups who are meant to help, let you down instead.

Children who have endured abuse need to have these experiences acknowledged by a therapist. Of course, this is just a first step and does not mean that the therapist cannot go on to interpret distortions that arise in the context of the abuse or identifications with the abuser.

Polly (Chapter 7), who was abandoned by her own mother and then a series of foster mothers, tried to distort her need for a mother by telling herself she could get by without emotional dependence. She felt she could secretly manipulate adults who would not notice her detachment and subversion of their care. The latter, harsher interpretation of her motives has to be put in context of the earlier devastating deprivation if it is to be balanced. It is this balance between one's compassion for the victim and one's toughness toward the destructive aspects of self that is particularly hard to get across. Children with horrible childhoods tend to pick up and magnify the negative in what is said to them. Anne Alvarez (1983) has advocated interpretations that lean toward a positive rather than a negative ending. Rather than 'you believe that I will abandon you because you are angry and jealous', it may be better to say, 'because you experience all those angry and jealous feelings, it makes it hard for you to believe I can want to come back'. The difference between these seemingly equivalent sentences can be immense. A child may hardly hear the first three words 'you believe that' and only hear damning words about themselves. This is what they expect and believe. The second interpretation cannot be easily distorted to a negative. The fact that this interpretation may not be believed is probable but that is different from hearing oneself condemned and discarded. It is difficult to grasp how negatively and with what hostility and despair, disordered children will approach an encounter offered as therapy. This is the more difficult to appreciate when the child does not say so directly but may be silent or distract attention from the real issue by fussing about an incidental one. Surely a good therapist will pick all this up in the transference and counter-transference? Well, eventually when one is close enough not to be misled. I look back on my early work in this field, however, and feel that I was blind.

I consistently underrated the abusive experiences of the children I met and it was hard to be uncondemning when they were persistently destructive. Locating all of the keys to their behaviour in the past is to turn them into pitiful victims but does not help them find a way forward. Recognising their own power to destroy and disrupt gives them back some agency in their lives and the need to understand and control themselves. However, if we demand that these children take responsibility for their actions, it must be with understanding and tolerance for how they have come to survive. If we can bear to know about their abuse and still help them toward different survival strategies they can help themselves to bridge that gap. Where we polarise and split the different aspects of the child we are ourselves resorting to defensive manoeuvres.

Working with others to contain such young people is the best way to keep more hopeful outcomes alive. This is work that can make therapists, social workers and carers either 'burned-out' and defeated or omnipotent and unrealistic. The load needs to be shared. In child and adolescent mental health services (CAMHS), therapy for fostered children should be a two-professional case. One therapist attends to the inner world of the child, the other concentrates on the network. Liaison of the therapeutic duo can function as a parental couple who hold the child's development in mind between them. In settings where I have worked outside CAMHS as a uni-professional, I have sought to make a strong partnership with the allocated social worker. If this partnership works well, therapy usually holds together and results in improvement. Where it fails it becomes extremely hard to come to a positive result. Sometimes the partners can be foster carer and therapist and I have had successful outcomes with this arrangement.

Too often it seems, budgetary concerns of health and social services conspire to deny the dreadful emotional condition of this population of children. For too long we professionals have become inured to the fact that chronically disordered children are being given inadequate mental health care. We do not accept it for physical ailments. Imagine a system of health care where only accident and emergency treatment was available: no treatment for chronic conditions, no heart surgery, no chemotherapy, no treatments longer than twelve weeks. Why do we accept these sorts of models for mental disorders in children?

The children in these pages have long-standing conditions and many are chronically disordered with poor prognosis. Is it extraordinary to predict that it may take two or three years to get them well?

I have contrasted elsewhere (Hunter 1999), the cost of individual psychotherapy with the cost of residential communities for children in care. If a child in a foster home can receive therapy two or three times a week there is often a real chance to keep the placement going. I am concerned that pressure to deliver cheaper treatment and failure to bear the cost of outcome research has resulted in psychotherapists' failure to advance this model of treatment. Are we guilty of watering down our treatment plan to a point of inefficacy?

Where children are held in supported foster care programmes, and are reliably brought to weekly therapy, it is possible to effect a good outcome in once-per-week treatment if it can be sustained for a number of years. Where a child is very distressed or distressing, or cannot be predicted to stay in placement longer than one year, it is preferable to see them at least twice each week. In practice once-weekly therapy results in much longer gaps between sessions. There are up to 12 weeks interrupted by holidays. There will be minor illnesses of the child, therapist and foster carer which result in cancellation. In effect once-weekly treatment averages out at 35 sessions over a year. Twice-weekly therapy, by contrast, means that it is rare not to see the child every week excepting holidays. Illnesses rarely occupy more than two or three days in a week so usually one session is still attended.

Again, the younger the child the shorter the breaks between sessions need to be. It really is a tall order for a 5-year-old to wait a week to finish an important confidence. Where one overstretches the child's capacity to connect one session to another it may be impossible to defeat the overwhelming sense of fragmentation. The more slowly therapy advances the longer in years may be needed to bring resolution of inner conflicts. Thus Polly, in Chapter 7, had 3½ years of treatment. The worry on my part was that she would move away before we had resolved her identification with her abuser. It is arguable that more intensive work over the course of a year was a better strategy.

I have treated 'children in transition' and I am an advocate for the belief that 'something is better than nothing'. However, I would not like to minimise the difficulty of therapy in a context of uncertainty. It may mean that parts of the work cannot be completed. It may give too good an excuse to the young person to regard the therapist as untrustworthy. Psychotherapy within a long-term care plan is likely to be much more therapeutic.

I have intended this book to be a 'warts and all' account of the practice of psychotherapy with looked-after children. I hope it will raise as many questions as it has answered. During the course of this work I have met many children who had lost themselves in feelings that they did not acknowledge or control. I have wanted to play a part in finding them and enabling them to find their way.

Glossary

adhesive relationship, adhesive identification Esther Bick (1964: 558) coined the term adhesive identification. It applies to an indiscriminate, rapid and superficial attachment. The child tries to desperately attach him- or herself to the therapist by copying them, trying to merge with the therapist in order to defend themselves from the terror of being alone. The child may feel so identified with the therapist that they use their gestures and phrases and may believe that they actually possess all of the therapist's abilities and qualities.

Asperger's syndrome, autism Asperger's syndrome is a psychiatric term used in the *International Classification of Diseases*. It is a milder form of autism.

Autism is diagnosed where a child has early-onset severe social communication difficulties together with restricted interests and odd mannerisms of an obsessive nature. These children cannot translate social cues and meanings. They cannot empathise, and fail to recognise emotions or respond to feelings appropriately. Most autistic children are mentally retarded and limited in their use of language.

Asperger's syndrome describes higher-functioning autistic children or those who have some but not all of the autistic features. Higher IQ and language development probably allows such children to find routes to develop social behaviours whilst the underlying failure to empathise remains.

Severe early deprivation is known to result in autistic features that are responsive to change in better circumstances and with help.

attachment patterns In infancy these are classifiable as:

- secure: uses caregiver as a secure base and plays and explores in their presence. At separation may or may not show distress but greets positively on reunion, seeks comfort if upset and returns to play and exploration;

- avoidant: seems uninterested in caregiver, explores busily and shows little distress at separation. Ignores or avoids caregiver on reunion;
- resistant/ambivalent: minimal exploration, preoccupied with caregiver, unsettled. After separation both seeks and resists contact, very angry or very passive;
- disorganised/disoriented: in the caregiver's presence behaviour is disorganised or odd e.g. frozen watchfulness.

attention deficit hyperactivity disorder, ADHD This controversial condition is a clinical diagnosis and therefore subject to interpretation and clinical judgement. ICD-10 specifies that it must involve marked restlessness, inattentiveness and impulsiveness allowing for the child's mental and chronological age. The condition must be pervasive across different settings such as home and school. Early onset, before 7 years, and persistence of the condition beyond 6 months are also required for the diagnosis. Anxiety, emotional disorders and post-traumatic stress have to be differentiated from ADHD.

Stimulant medication, methylphenidate, is commonly used to control ADHD in childhood.

borderline personality disorder Different definitions of this term are legion but Fonagy *et al.* (1995) refer to Gunderson's (1984) helpful criteria which include adult impulsivity, low achievement, heightened affectivity, manipulative suicide attempts, mild psychotic experiences and disturbed interpersonal relationships.

Care Order A legal order under the Children Act 1989. This places the child in the care of a named local authority which assumes parental responsibility for the child and acquires the power to determine how far others shall be allowed to exercise their parental responsibility.

Children Act 1989 A major framework of current child-care legislation, this Act refers amongst other things to the welfare of the child, which shall be the court's paramount consideration (i.e. beyond any claim of other interests or parents' rights). Section 31(2) establishes 'a court may only make a care order or supervision order if it is satisfied that the child concerned is suffering or is likely to suffer significant harm'. The Act also seeks to balance the harm that may be done by admission to public care compared to the harm of leaving the child with its family. Other principles in this Act are the principles of keeping family links intact as far as possible so that siblings are to be placed together, accommodation with relatives is preferred to substitute care, parents are to be enabled to remain involved and parental responsibilities are never withdrawn.

containment The process of absorbing emotional processes or of integrating emotions. A father can be said to be containing toward his child if he perceives and responds to her distress in a feeling and measured way. A person is said to be contained when they can balance and integrate conflicting and ambivalent feelings without resorting to defence mechanisms.

counter-transference Those feelings which are evoked in the therapist as a direct response to the child's transference. For example, children transfer their feelings of deprivation from a neglectful parent onto the therapist. Counter-transference feelings of guilt may be evoked in the therapist.

defence mechanisms These are psychological processes or manoeuvres by which the self protects itself from the knowledge of anxiety or conflicting emotions. Originally used by Freud in a more technical way, the term is broadly used in this book to mean any defensive conscious or unconscious process which is used to ward off painful feelings.

dissociation A defence related to splitting. A person can be in a dissociated state when they are out of touch with feelings or memories that cause anxiety to a traumatic degree. Dissociation is detachment not because the pain has been integrated but because it has been split off from consciousness.

DSM-IV *Diagnostic and Statistical Manual of the American Psychiatric Association* is an American version, not identical to the WHO classifications. Those who are interested in current diagnostic issues in child psychiatry should refer to Goodman and Scott (1997) for a plain and simple introduction to the field.

flashback An intensely vivid memory of a traumatic experience that returns repeatedly.

ICD-10 *International Classification of Diseases of the World Health Organisation*, tenth edition, is a manual of clinical descriptions and diagnostic guidelines for the use of mental health professionals as an aid to diagnosis.

interpretation Making unconscious things conscious by talking about them. Therapists interpret unconscious anxieties and defences against anxiety. Interpretation can be located in the transference relationship between therapist and child or within the psychological world of the child. However, a useful way to get near to interpretation in highly defended children is to locate the therapist's insight in real relationships the child has had with others. Alternatively, I find that children who are too scared or defended to tolerate these insights can accept interpretation in terms of their play. It is less threatening for them to admit that a play character is greedy, for example, than to admit that they are greedy. This can be used as a halfway stage to accepting these motives as their own.

introjection A normal developmental process of psychologically taking in external important people, attitudes, relationships and events. A child introjects his mother and father and takes in their qualities as he has perceived and experienced them. Introjection is a necessary precondition for identification.

looked-after children Children are 'looked after' when they are either in care by virtue of a formal order made by a court or are provided with accommodation through a voluntary arrangement under the Act. Further information can be found in the usefully clear text of Butler and Roberts (1997).

manic defence, manic activity These refer to hurried, controlling attitudes and actions with denial of anxiety and a claim to omnipotence. There is often an identification with powerful people. Children using manic defences cover up their vulnerability and feelings of powerlessness with inflated ideas of their strength and ability.

manic reparation A child may loosen her/his defences sufficiently to allow the thought that someone has been hurt or damaged but believes she/he can alone (and by omnipotent control) fix the problem.

object, good object–bad object This word invariably means a person, not a thing. It is used in the sense of 'object of desire', a target or a source. Early on, children struggle with ambivalence and tend to relate to important others as 'all good' or 'all bad' according to their current feeling.

Oedipus complex The boy child's fantasy that he is a partner to his mother, sexually and emotionally and therefore a rival to his father. Oedipus in the Greek tragedy slept with his mother and killed his father. The girl child's fantasy is equivalent: that she is her father's partner and her mother's rival.

Kleinian psychotherapists view this constellation as only one of a number of similar fantasies, namely the wish to be the mother rather than partner her, the boy's longing to bear children, the girl's wish to have a penis, the child's denial that adults are more mature than children, etc.

parental couple Refers to the concept that mother and father are supportive partners, sexually and emotionally, and are independent grown-ups. The child must adjust to odd-man-out status, however loved and wanted he is.

post-traumatic stress disorder, PTSD This is defined by the experience, for longer than one month, of symptoms that involve:

- re-experience of the trauma via flashbacks, intrusive thoughts, re-enactments in play or dreams;
- avoidance of certain situations or things connected with the trauma or numbing of responses to such events;
- increased arousal, hyper-vigilance or irritability.

projection The attribution to another of wishes and feelings that are one's own. Projection is also assumed to be a necessary developmental process: the infant projects its rage or fear away from itself and into the mother. The infant introjects an idea of the mother distorted by its own projections. Therefore the baby may fear mother may eat him as he wished to devour her. He may then split this frightening thought and keep an idea of a gentle feeding mother whilst he fears that a bogeyman will eat him.

projective identification Used here in the sense of a very strong and primitive form of projection which needs to be lodged with the therapist in order for the child to feel received. The therapist has to identify with the projection in order to empathise adequately with the child.

reparation True reparation always involves the child's:

- acknowledgement of their own anger, aggression or destructiveness;
- the limits of their ability to destroy;
- the limits of their ability to mend or put right the person or situation;
- an acknowledgement that another adult can help redress the harm.

The prototypical scenario is the child realises he attacked his mother, the harm done is limited, he alone is not responsible for mother's well-being, his father looks after his mother. He realises he is a child in relation to a parental couple.

splitting A way of defending oneself from ambivalent and therefore uncomfortable emotions is to split them so that they are assigned to different objects or so that they are strictly separated in the mind.

A person can 'split' their angry feelings from their loving feelings by feeling only one at a time. A child who loves and hates his mother says 'I love my mum, it's you I hate' to a foster mother.

transference In psychotherapy this term applies to specific aspects of the patient–therapist relationship: those aspects that are transferred from the infantile part of the self which related to a parent in this way. The situation of seeking help from a therapist in an intimate one-to-one setting invokes patterns of interaction and feelings that attended the infant–mother and infant–father relationship. Therapy is therefore the conscious use of the transference relationship.

unconscious Thoughts, feelings and mental processes of which a person is unaware are said to be unconscious. In therapy the emphasis is on a person's motives for repressing thoughts and motives for distracting oneself from such knowledge.

Freud and others tended to imagine the unconscious as a deep and hidden place in the mind. Conflict and hidden agendas make unconscious meanings difficult to discover. Nevertheless, some of what is unconscious to the host can be obvious to another person, partly because we are inside ourselves and cannot easily see ourselves from the outside.

Training schools of child psychotherapy

The Association of Child Psychotherapists is the accrediting authority for child psychotherapy training recognised by the Department of Health. The recognised training schools are:

The Anna Freud Centre
21 Maresfield Gardens
Hampstead
London NW3 5SH
Tel: 020 7794 2313
Fax: 020 7794 6506

The Society of Analytical Psychotherapy
1 Daleham Gardens
London NW3 5BY
Tel: 020 7435 7696
Fax: 020 7431 1495

The Tavistock & Portman NHS Trust
The Tavistock Clinic
120 Belsize Lane
London NW3 5BA
Tel: 020 7435 7111
Fax: 020 7791 8741

The British Association of Psychotherapists
37 Mapesbury Road
London NW2 7HJ
Tel: 020 8452 9823
Fax: 020 8452 5182

Birmingham Trust for Psychoanalytic Psychotherapy
Selly Oak Colleges
Elmfield House
998 Bristol Road
Birmingham B29 6LQ
Tel: 0121 472 4231

The Scottish Institute of Human Relations
13 Park Terrace
Glasgow G3 6BY
Tel: 0141 332 0011

References

Ainsworth, M. and Wittig, B. A. (1969) 'Attachment and the exploratory behaviour of one-year-olds in a strange situation', in B. M. Foss (ed.), *Determinants of Infant Behaviour, Vol. 4*, pp. 113–36, London: Methuen.

Ainsworth, M.D.S., Blehar, M., Waters, E. and Wall, S. (1978) *Patterns of Attachment*, Hillsdale, NJ: Lawrence Erlbaum Associates.

Alvarez, A. (1983) 'Problems in the use of counter-transference: getting it across', *Journal of Child Psychotherapy*, Vol. 9, No. 1.

Alvarez, A. (1985) 'The problem of neutrality: some reflections on the psychoanalytic attitude in the treatment of borderline and psychotic children', *Journal of Child Psychotherapy*, Vol. 11, No. 1, 87–104.

Alvarez, A. (1992) *Live Company*, London and New York: Tavistock/ Routledge.

American Psychiatric Association (1994) Diagnostic and Statistical Manual of Mental Disorders, 4th edn, DSM-IV. Washington DC: American Psychiatric Association.

Berelowitz, M. and Horne, A. (1992) 'Child mental health and the legacy of child guidance', *Association for Child Psychology and Psychiatry Review* Vol. 15, No. 1, 214–18.

Bick, E. (1964) 'Notes on infant observation in psychoanalytic training', *International Journal of Psychoanalysis*, Vol. 45, 558–66.

Bion, W. R. (1971) 'Container and contained', in *Attention and Interpretation*, London: Tavistock.

Bolton, D., O'Ryan, D., Udwin, O., Boyle, S. and Yule, W. (2000) 'The long term psychological effects of a disaster experienced in adolescence', *Journal of Child Psychology and Psychiatry*, Vol. 41, No. 4, 513–23.

Boston, M. and Szur, R. (1983) *Psychotherapy with Severely Deprived Children*, London: Karnac Books.

Breggin, M. (1997) *Brain Disabling Treatments in Psychiatry: Drugs, Electroshock and the Role of the FDA*, New York: Springer.

Butler, I. and Roberts, G. (1997) *Social Work with Children and Families – Getting into Practice*, London and Philadelphia: Jessica Kingsley.

Conners, C.K. (1995) *The Conners Rating Scales: Instruments for the Assessment of Childhood Psychopathology*, North Tonawanda, NY: Multi Health System.

DuPaul, G. J., Barkley, R. A. and McMurray, B. (1994) 'Response of children to methylphenidate: interaction with internalizing symptoms', *Journal of the American Academy of Child and Adolescent Psychiatry*, Vol.33, 894–903.

Farmer, E. and Pollock, S. (1998) 'Sexually abused and abusing children in substitute care', in *Caring for Children Away from Home: Messages from Research*, Chichester: Wiley/Department of Health.

Fonagy, P., Steele, M., Steele, H., Higgit, A. and Target, M. (1992) 'The theory and practice of resilience', *Journal of Child Psychology and Psychiatry*, Vol. 37, No. 2, 231–57.

Fonagy, P., Steele, M., Steele, H., Leigh, T., Kennedy, R., Mattoon, G. and Target, M. (1995) 'Attachment, the reflective self and borderline states: the predictive specificity of the adult attachment interview and pathological emotional development', in S. Goldberg, R. Muir and J. Kerr (eds), *Attachment Theory: Social Developmental and Clinical Perspectives*, London: The Analytic Press.

Freud, S. (1973) 'Anxiety and instinctual life', in *New Introductory Lectures on Psycho-Analysis*, J. Strachey (ed.) [first published in the Standard Edition, Vol. XXII, 1964] Harmondsworth: Penguin.

Furman, R. (1996) 'Methylphenidate and ADHD in Europe and the USA', in *Journal of Child Psychiatry*, Vol. 22, No. 1, 157–60.

Gaber, I. and Aldridge, J. (eds) (1994) *In the Best Interests of the Child: Culture, Identity and Transracial Adoption*, London: Free Association Books.

Goldberg, S., Muir, R. and Kerr, J. (eds) (1995) *Attachment Theory: Social, Developmental and Clinical Perspectives*, London: The Analytical Press.

Goodman, R. and Scott, S. (1997) *Child Psychiatry*, London: Blackwell Science.

Gunderson, J.G. (1984) *Borderline Personality Disorder*, Washington DC: American Psychiatric Press.

Green, B.L., Grace, M., Vary, M.G., Kramer, T.L., Gleser, G.C., and Leonard, A.C. (1994) 'Children of disaster in the second decade: A 17 year follow up of Buffalo Creek survivors', *Journal of the American Academy of Child and Adolescent Psychiatry*, Vol. 33, 71–9.

Henry, G. (1974) 'Doubly deprived', *Journal of Child Psychotherapy*, Vol. 4, No. 2, 29–43.

Hodges, J., Williams, B., Andreou, C., Lanyado, M., Bentovim, A. and Skuse, D. (1997) 'Children who sexually abuse other children', in Justice Wall (ed.) *Rooted Sorrows: Psychoanalytic Perspectives on Child Protection*, Bristol: Family Law.

Hopkins, J. (1990) 'The observed infant of attachment theory', *British Journal of Psychiatry*, Vol. 6, 460–71.

Hunter, M. (1993a) 'The emotional needs of children in care: an overview of 30 cases', *Association of Child Psychology and Psychiatry Review*, Vol. 15, No. 5, 214–18.

Hunter, M. (1993b) 'Working with the past', *Adoption and Fostering*, Vol. 17, No. 1: 31–6.

Hunter, M. (1999) 'The child and adolescent psychotherapist in the community', in M. Lanyado and A. Horne (eds), *The Handbook of Child and Adolescent Psychotherapy*, London and New York: Routledge.

Klein, M. (1975) *Love, Guilt and Reparation and Other Works 1921–1945*, London: Hogarth Press.

Lanyado, M. and Horne, A. (eds) (1999) *The Handbook of Child and Adolescent Psychotherapy*, London: Routledge.

Main, M. (1991) 'Metacognitive knowledge, metacognitive monitoring and singular (coherent) vs multiple (incoherent) model of attachment', in C. M. Parkes, J. Stevenson-Hinde and P. Marris (eds), *Attachment Across the Life Cycle*, London and New York: Routledge.

Matier, K., Halperin, J. M., Sharma, U. Newcorn, J. H. and Sathaye, N. (1992) 'Methylphenidate response in aggressive and non-aggressive ADHD children', *Journal of the American Academy of Child and Adolescent Psychiatry*, Vol. 31, 219–25.

Mrazek, P. B. and Kempe, C. H. (eds) (1987) *Sexually Abused Children and their Families*, Oxford: Pergamon Press.

Mullen, P., Martin, J., Anderson, J., Romans, S. and Herbison, G. (1993) 'Childhood sexual abuse and mental health in adult life', *British Journal of Psychiatry*, Vol. 163, 721–32.

Ogden, T. (1979) 'On projective identification', *International Journal of Psychoanalysis*, Vol. 60, 357–73.

Orford, E. (1998) 'Wrestling with the whirlwind: an approach to the understanding of ADD/ADHD', *Journal of Child Psychotherapy*, Vol. 24, No. 2, 253–66.

Overmeyer, S. and Taylor E. (1999) 'Annotation: principles of treatment for hyperkinetic disorder', *Journal of Child Psychology and Psychiatry*, Vol. 40, No. 8, 1147–57.

Parkes, C. M., Stevenson-Hinde, J. and Marris, P. (eds) (1991) *Attachment Across the Life Cycle*, London and New York: Routledge.

Perry, B., Pollard, R., Blakley, T., Baker, W., Vigilante, D. (1995) 'Childhood trauma, the neurobiology of adaptation and use dependent development of the brain: how states become traits', *Infant Mental Health Journal*, Vol. 16, No, 4, 271–91.

Piaget, J. (1954) *The Construction of Reality in the Child*, New York: Basic Books.

Pliszka, S. R., Borcherding, S. H., Spratley, K. Leon, S. and Irick, S. (1997) 'Measuring inhibitory control in children', *Journal of Developmental and Behavioral Pediatrics*, Vol. 18, 254–9.

Rutter, M. (1982) 'Syndrome attributed to minimal brain dysfunction', *Journal of Psychiatry*, Vol. 139, 21–33.

Sandler, A. M. (1985) 'On interpretation and holding', *Journal of Child Psychotherapy*, Vol. 11, No. 1, 3–15.

Segal, H. (1979) 'The play technique', in *Klein*, Modern Masters series, London: Fontana.

Sinason, V. (ed.) (1998) *Memory in Dispute*, London: Karnac.

Stoller, R. J. (1986) *Perversion: The Erotic Form of Hatred*, London: Karnac.

Tannock, R. (1998) 'Attention deficit hyperactivity disorder: advances in cognitive neurobiological and genetic research', in *Journal of Child Psychology and Psychiatry*, Vol. 39, No. 1, Annual Research Review: 65–100.

Tannock, R. Ickowicz, A. and Schachar, R. (1995) 'Differential effects of methylphenidate on working memory in ADHD children with and without comorbid anxiety', *Journal of the American Academy of Child and Adolescent Psychiatry*, Vol. 34, 886–96.

Urman, R. Ickowitz, A. Fulford, P. and Tannock, R. (1995) 'An exaggerated cardiovascular response to methylphenidate in ADHD children with anxiety', *Journal of Child and Adolescent Psychopharmacology*, Vol. 5, 29–37.

Van der Kolk, B. (1996) 'Trauma and memory', in Van der Kolk, B., McFarlane, A.C. and Weisaeth, L. (eds) *Traumatic Stress*, New York: Guilford Press.

van Ijzendoorn, M. H. (1995) 'Adult attachment representations, parental responsiveness and infant attachment: a meta-analysis on the predictive validity of the Adult Attachment Interview', *Psychological Bulletin*, Vol. 117, 387–403.

Wade, J., Biehal, N., Clayden, J. and Stein, M. (1998) 'Going missing: young people absent from care', in *Caring for Children Away from Home: Messages from Research*, Chichester: Wiley/Department of Health.

Widener, A.J. (1998) 'Beyond Ritalin: the importance of therapeutic work with parents and children diagnosed ADD/ADHD', *Journal of Child Psychotherapy*, Vol. 24, No. 2, 267–81.

Winnicott, D. (1965) *The Maturational Process and the Facilitating Environment*, London: Hogarth Press.

World Health Organization (1993) *The ICD-10 Classification of Mental and Behavioural Disorders: Diagnostic Criteria for Research*. Geneva: World Health Organization.

Yule, W., Udwin, O. and Murdoch, K. (1990) 'The Jupiter sinking: effects on children's fears, depression and anxiety', *Journal of Child Psychology and Psychiatry*, Vol. 31, 1051–61.

Index

Printed in the United States
by Baker & Taylor Publisher Services